An Autism Casebook for Parents and Practitioners

Drawing from the author's extensive clinical experience, this autism casebook offers stimulating reflections and a fresh perspective on how we assess, diagnose and ultimately treat young children thought to be autistic.

Challenging what she perceives as the rampant over-diagnosis and misdiagnosis of autism, and the commonly accepted status of autism as an unchangeable trait, Dr. Levin Fox illustrates how the developmental play strategies of DIRFloortime, combined with the creative psychological perspective of Reuven Feuerstein, create an effective way of identifying the child's strengths behind the autistic symptoms. The chapters are an accessible mix of clinical insights, theoretical reflections and vivid case stories that argue and illustrate that qualitative assessment methods based on play have the power to yield a more accurate clinical understanding of a child's difficulties—and strengths—than conventional symptom-focused autism assessment methods.

This engaging casebook will stimulate practitioners, educators and students in the field of autism to question commonly held assumptions when assessing and treating autistic children, as it both urges and illustrates more reflective practice. Parents of children considered autistic will find renewed encouragement and hope in these enlightening case stories.

Shoshana Levin Fox, EdD, is a child psychologist specializing in play therapy. Since completing doctoral studies in Canada, she has worked in Jerusalem, where she lives with her husband.

An Autism Casebook for Parents and Practitioners

The Child Behind the Symptoms

Shoshana Levin Fox

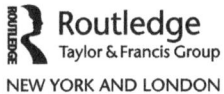
Routledge
Taylor & Francis Group

NEW YORK AND LONDON

First published 2021
by Routledge
52 Vanderbilt Avenue, New York, NY 10017

and by Routledge
2 Park Square, Milton Park, Abingdon, Oxon, OX14 4RN

Routledge is an imprint of the Taylor & Francis Group, an informa business

Library of Congress Cataloging-in-Publication Data
Names: Fox, Shoshana Levin, author.
Title: An autism casebook for parents and practitioners : the child
behind the symptoms / Shoshana Levin Fox.
Description: New York, NY : Routledge, 2021.| Includes
bibliographical references and index. Identifiers: LCCN 2020030038
(print) | LCCN 2020030039 (ebook) | ISBN 9780367434434
(hardback) | ISBN 9780367434410 (paperback) | ISBN
9781003003250 (ebook)
Subjects: LCSH: Autism in children—Case studies. | Autistic
children—Case studies. | Autistic children—Rehabilitation—Case
studies. | Parents of autistic children—Case studies.
Classification: LCC RJ506.A9 F683 2021 (print) | LCC RJ506.A9
(ebook) | DDC 618.92/85882—dc23
LC record available at https://lccn.loc.gov/2020030038
LC ebook record available at https://lccn.loc.gov/2020030039

ISBN: 978-0-367-43443-4 (hbk)
ISBN: 978-0-367-43441-0 (pbk)
ISBN: 978-1-003-00325-0 (ebk)

Typeset in Baskerville
by MPS Limited, Dehradun

To all my teachers, young and old

Contents

Acknowledgments

The contributions and talents of so many mentors, colleagues and friends resound within this book that I will surely fail in acknowledging them all. To those whose handprints were visible and whose heartbeats were audible in helping so many children over the years, but whose names I have overlooked, I apologize profusely for the oversight.

Thank you so much…

To John Allan for guiding me so warmly and wisely in the use of play, to the late Ian Kent Eckstein for his deep commitment to caring and truth, and to the late Reuven Feuerstein for his brilliance, courage and inspiration.

To Rafael Feuerstein for his encouragement.

To the Feuerstein Institute's remarkable team of talented and devoted professionals that over the years included so many wonderful colleagues and friends: Sari Aloni, Bruria Amichai, Tehila Amedi, Gili Amorai, Moshe Avital, Orit Berkovitz, Batya Cohen, Ayelet Eitan, Chaya Ginton, Steven Gross, Chana Nakav, Monica Paz, Adina Rathner, Revital Rubin, Naama Saffer, Rina Schreiber, Tracey Stevens, Leahle Weiss and so many more amazing people. I learned from you all.

To friends and warm colleagues Deborah Court, Allan Gonsher, Ilene Lee and Alisa Vig, for your critical reading of portions of this book and for your helpful comments and support. Your voices echo in these pages as well.

Heartfelt, to my husband Shlomo, for encouraging me to climb the mountain of writing this book and who, steadfast and true, held my hand along the upward path.

To the Almighty, for the gift of this life and the opportunity to give.

Foreword

My late father, Professor Reuven Feuerstein, pioneered groundbreaking techniques based on the assumed modifiability of human functioning. His ideas improved significantly the quality of life of countless children and adults with special needs. Just at the time Professor Feuerstein was looking to expand the range of his work with autistic children, the author of this unique autism casebook, Shoshana Levin Fox, joined the Feuerstein Institute. Working with an exceptional group of colleagues from a variety of disciplines, Shoshana brought to the Institute her expertise from the field of play therapy and proceeded to apply her understanding of play in child development to her special interest in autism.

The results for the children were very good. As she grew in appreciating the value of using play to assess and treat autistic children, Shoshana began to share her knowledge and experience with visiting professionals at our workshops in Israel and abroad and, of course, with the parents of the children she treated. Now in this spirited casebook, she shares with her readers the essence of what she learned and applied over the years about autism and its diagnosis and about the power of the dynamic assessment of autism. Her treatment interventions always kept the focus on the individual's potential for modifiability, the concept that lies at the heart of the work at the Feuerstein Institute, which I now head.

I found this absorbing autism casebook to be an honest one. Shoshana shares the journey toward many successful outcomes, but she does not shy away from talking about disappointments or even those rarer failures. Through the case narratives, she invites the reader to join her in her office with the children and also to join her in questioning many aspects of assessment and intervention that are often taken for granted in the field of autism. So there are more than stories here. There are questions, reflections and challenges to professional practice related to autism. There is also much that is practical and down-to-earth, as she shares with parents and professionals the ideas, activities and recommendations that made a difference in her clients' lives.

Without sacrificing the integrity of either worldview, Shoshana combined aspects of Professor Feuerstein's approach with the elements of

DIRFloortime. Professionals will find within this book intellectually stimulating observations. They will also hear in it a call for increasingly reflective practice. Parents will feel supported, since assisting parents was such an important part of the work. Even when she wrestles with challenging theoretical issues related to the cases described, her writing remains clear and coherent, so that any reader can follow and understand the ideas fully. The depth of the discussion is maintained without the language becoming convoluted. It is gratifying to me that I encouraged Shoshana to write about her clinical experiences and that the result is a truly enjoyable and stimulating contribution to professional literature in the field of autism.

Rafael S. Feuerstein
President, Feuerstein Institute, Jerusalem

Introduction
A Call from the Trenches

From time to time throughout my career working with special needs and typically developing children, I would be offered an administrative, consultative or teaching position. Though sometimes tempted, I usually declined, explaining that I preferred to continue working in the trenches: with the children, grappling with their difficulties, attempting along with my colleagues to wrest the maximum potential from within each child. Over the past roughly twenty-five years, I encountered in those trenches hundreds, even thousands, of children, the majority of whom had been diagnosed as "autistic" or a related clinical synonym before they entered the doors of my workplace.

Autism is a powerful word. It is a charged diagnosis capable of shaking the confidence of the most loving parents. It is a diagnosis which carries with it an ominous sense of an innate condition whose symptoms, it is widely thought, may perhaps be treated and improved, but for which dramatic change in a child's essence should not be anticipated. It is a diagnosis whose impact is growing exponentially as the number of children being diagnosed as autistic continues to proliferate. And the research race is on to determine genetic markers for autism, as well as brain functioning and brain structural differences between typical and autistic populations. One encounters new information about autism, its inferred causes and its treatment, almost daily in the press. Yet not all that can be said about autism has been written. There is more that needs to be said from a different perspective, and hence the stories of the children in this book.

My clinical experience over the past generation, along with that of my colleagues, challenges many of the accepted "givens" about autism so prevalent in the field. The reader will encounter strong undercurrents within the case studies in this book, namely, my concerns that autism is being widely misdiagnosed and over-diagnosed, and that the preconception of autism as an incurable trait is harmful to the prognosis of many children so misdiagnosed (and even to those who have been correctly diagnosed).

Effective, proactive, play-based and creative ways of therapeutically working with children who are thought to be autistic do exist. This book does not claim to have discovered the "only way" to reach and meaningfully help autistic children. However, if the responses by many visiting professionals to our lectures over the years offer any gauge, in our work we do appear to have stumbled upon, no, forged a qualitatively different way of viewing and assessing autism. This way of viewing autism is not simply refreshing. It has proven essential and even life-saving in its capacity to detect strengths in the child which have been obscured rather than clarified by the current hyper-elastic criteria of the autism diagnosis. A qualitative, functionally descriptive way of playfully entering into the labyrinth of a child's symptoms with the aim of discovering developmental strengths has proven incredibly useful in revealing the true children behind the autistic symptoms.

The reader may already have noticed that I have avoided using the term "autistic spectrum," assumed today to hold clinical relevance. Another undercurrent within this volume: with the onset of the term "autistic spectrum," I worry that practitioners have seriously compromised the ability to diagnose differentially and to comprehend the individual weaknesses—and strengths—of young children who present with complex social communication difficulties.

Between 1992 and 2017, I had the privilege of working with special children at a special place alongside its special staff. This book relates the stories of some of the children with whom I worked. In 1992 I had just completed a doctorate in counseling psychology, with a subspecialty in play therapy, under the mentorship of John Allan at the University of British Columbia. Thirty days after my doctoral defense, I was boarding a plane for Israel, with a postdoctoral fellowship in hand, planning to carry out a research project in autism at the Feuerstein Institute, headed by world-renowned psychologist Professor Reuven Feuerstein. I already possessed a career-long interest in the subject of autism, stretching back nearly fifteen years before that fateful flight. In various early career positions in the fields of education and psychology I had often worked with children diagnosed as autistic. That interest was about to intensify.

A word about the special place alluded to above. Known familiarly as "the Institute," the Feuerstein Institute was founded by Sorbonne-educated psychologist Reuven Feuerstein and actively guided and headed by him until his death in 2014, a few months before his ninety-third birthday. The afternoon he died he told one of his staff that he wanted to discuss his concerns about a certain young adult with special needs in a few hours' time, but that he was tired and needed first to rest. He never woke up from that nap. Not surprisingly to those of us who had the privilege of working alongside him, struggling to keep up with his grueling, devoted and inspired pace, Reuven died with his boots on.

The Professor, or just simply Reuven, as he was affectionately known by staff, families, children and by leading specialists worldwide in the fields of education, psychology, child development, neurology and others, was a larger than life personality. He was brilliant, with a mastery not only of many languages but also more pertinently with a deep understanding of such topics as genetic syndromes, pediatric neurology, psychiatry, autism, brain plasticity—long before the term was coined—and more. He was courageous. The fields of education and psychology are heavy with accepted truisms, which for the Professor were neither automatically accepted nor necessarily true. There were no sacred cows for the Professor. A developmental diagnosis like autism, in his estimation, might possibly serve as a weak hypothesis for the condition of a child, but it more often than not clouded our insight, masking the complex roots of a child's problem while at the same time obscuring the latent energy and positive abilities within the child that could help symptoms considered intransigent (or innate) to fade.

Modifiability, the inherent capacity of the human being to change, was the watchword of the many cognitive enhancement and learning potential materials he developed throughout his lifetime. Those materials, chief among them the Learning Potential Assessment Device (LPAD),[1] a qualitative, interactive method of determining children's and adults' potential to think and grow rather than quantifying their cognitive performance, and the cognitive development booklets known as Feuerstein's Instrumental Enrichment (FIE)[2] are used worldwide in dozens of countries. Their effectiveness has been documented by scores of research studies.[3,4,5] When the concept of the plasticity of the brain entered mainstream medicine and psychology in recent years, the Professor chuckled with delight. Without the benefit of superlative brain imaging technology, he had intuited the capacity of brain cells for growth and transformation two generations earlier.

With an alternative approach to psychology which focuses on latent cognitive potential and developmental growth rather than on pathology, with materials that are effective in ferreting out hidden strengths within children and adults whose latent abilities had been ill-served by conventional intelligence and developmental evaluations, and with a deep and inspired human being at its helm, the Institute was and is a very special place. It continues to draw from all over the world families of special needs children and adults who seek its assessment and therapeutic services. Children and adults with learning problems, physical disabilities, autism, brain injuries, genetic syndromes and complex inexplicable conditions continue to crowd the halls, waiting for assessment or therapeutic interventions rooted in his visionary approach.

His clinical insight, his deep humanity and his brilliance drew not only struggling and impaired populations, so many of whom were significantly helped by him and his staff. His work also attracted many therapists, educators and other specialists, like myself, hungry for a vision of psychology and education which stressed potential over pathology, and which provided a conceptual framework and tools for transforming what initially appears hopeless to hopeful.

Miracles, as they say, take longer. They did, but we all worked very hard and so we were privileged to see many: children who had been considered retarded learning to read and then integrate into regular schools, learning disabled children for whom the word "disabled" proved to be a misnomer, brain-injured children and adults whose progress stunned medical experts, and children who had been diagnosed elsewhere as autistic who improved beyond expectation. And when the miraculous was not achieved, in many cases significant and impressive progress was.

Before boarding that plane to Israel many years ago, friends had asked me what I anticipated doing at the Feuerstein Institute. I replied that I expected to have a little office from which I would carry out postdoctoral research comparing active, assertive play interventions with autistic children with conditions of accepting, empathic nondirective play therapy. I was wrong. When I arrived, there were not even enough offices in that former setting for staff members to assess and treat children. An office was out of the question. Nor was there adequate time to devote to careful research.

Soon there were competing demands on the time I had anticipated doing research. Professor Feuerstein immediately assigned me to assessing and treating children, in particular children who were considered autistic. Renowned for its pioneering work with Down syndrome children, the Feuerstein Institute was eager to deepen and broaden its involvement in the field of autism. So was I. My research project was carried out, though not under the most rigorous standards. Having just completed a doctorate specializing in nondirective play therapy with typical children, I was surprised to find that more proactive, energetic play approaches elicited better relationship and communication responses from the autistic children in the study than an approach of quiet empathic acceptance. It was a lesson that would be re-learned many hundreds of times in the years to come, with the many autistic children whom I assessed and treated.

At first I felt very much adrift at the Institute, out of my element, having just completed four years delving deeply into the world of affect, the inner emotional life of the child, and learning the wonderful treatment modality of play therapy. The Institute spoke the language of cognitive development. My heart was with the language of affect. It was the world of play which would bridge the two realms.

The Professor maintained active, warm relationships with many leading experts in the fields of education, psychology, neurology, child development and more. One of these individuals was Dr. Serena Wieder, co-developer with the late Dr. Stanley Greenspan of Floortime, a play-based, developmentally grounded intervention for autistic children, widely used and enjoying much success.[6,7] In the late 1990s and for several years following, Professor Feuerstein ensured that the nucleus of his staff who worked with autistic children were able to attend the remarkable international conferences on the topic of autism organized by Wieder and Greenspan. These conferences showcased medical research, findings about the effectiveness of their developmental (D), individually attuned (I), relationship based (R) model DIR,[8] state of the art information on topics related to nutrition, allergies, auditory processing and much more as related to autism, all presented by experts in their fields. Following one of these conferences, I flew again to the East Coast to take an initial course in the essentials of DIRFloortime practice. This was followed by several tutorial group workshops with Serena Wieder, which she conducted when in Israel.

With a strong background in play therapy, I was well aware of the critical importance of play in the development of the young child. One does not need to have training in play therapy in order to appreciate and apply the principles discussed in this book. One does require, however, a deep appreciation and understanding of how powerful a tool play can be in reaching any child. If we carefully observe children at play, we will find that, in their play, children are telling us so much about themselves in a myriad of developmental realms: their understanding of the world and of social relationships, their capacity for relating, their capacity for imagination and pretense, their capacity for language and communication, their capacity for the expression of emotions and for emotional reciprocity, their capacity for focus and attention, their levels of fine motricity (finger and hand dexterity) and gross motricity (larger bodily movements), their levels of understanding and cognition (thinking), their personality development and sense of self. Play truly functions as a mirror of the child's capacities. If we look deeply into that mirror, we find that so much is reflected about the developmental functioning of the child. The information we glean will not necessarily lead us to statistical information which can be normed, but it will provide us with a rich qualitative description of the difficulties—and capacities—of each child.

Play offers yet more. It is a two-way street. From one perspective, play *reflects and expresses* the child's challenges and abilities. From another, play offers an active, energetic *conduit to influence and improve* the child's abilities. To a remarkable degree, the developers of DIRFloortime utilized the power of active, energetic and even caringly intrusive play to pierce the autistic shell and to woo the autistic child into relationship and reciprocal communication.

I had been schooled to use play in play therapy as an empathically receptive tool, providing the emotional greenhouse conditions for troubled children to begin to trust, find their strengths and shed their symptoms. My general postdoctoral research findings, though, had shown that proactively asserting oneself into the world of the autistic child serves to elicit more positive responses than by empathically accepting the child (as in play therapy practice) and assuming that he or she will find the direction out of the autism labyrinth. To some readers this may be obvious. For me, it was part of a steep learning curve. Beyond these postdoctoral research findings, after having gained some competence in the playfully assertive strategies of DIRFloortime, my growing experience with autistic children at the Institute was confirming to me that proactive play strategies can work wonders in treating children considered autistic. Further, these same play strategies served me as a basis for carrying out qualitative (descriptive), interactive assessments of the functioning of children thought to be autistic.

Dynamic (interactive) assessments are the lifeblood of the work at the Institute. In a dynamic assessment, the assessor (or mediator in Feuerstein parlance) seeks change, evidence of modifiability, in cognitive and developmental abilities during the intentionally interactive assessment process itself. The dynamic assessor does not seek to quantify and then norm statistical evidence of a child's performance. Rather, in dynamic assessment the assessor seeks descriptive understanding of the child's process functioning and, above all, clues as to what aspects of the mediator's intentional and active intervention prompted the change in the child's profile in real time during the assessment.

Experience and comfort with play, play-based DIRFloortime strategies, and the need for qualitative assessment information in order to tease out the true potential of the child behind the autistic symptoms—it all began to come together. This book relates the impact of the synergistic use of play strategies derived from DIRFloortime during dynamic assessments (and treatment) within the Feuerstein clinical paradigm, which is dedicated to modifiability and the realization of the maximum potential of each child.

At its heart, this book is a casebook telling of the challenges, while charting the progress, of children who arrived at the Institute having been diagnosed elsewhere as autistic. The story of each child has much to teach: about the limits of a diagnostic term, about the dangers of misdiagnosis and overused diagnostic terminology, about how preconceptions about the intransigence of certain symptoms too often inhibit therapeutic efforts, about the developmental and therapeutic benefits of seeking strengths within the most challenging profile, about how play strategies can trump symptom lists in enlightening us about a child's potential, and about the developmental resilience of many children and the courage of their parents.

Following the first section of eight case stories, the second section presents the theoretical groundings of work that combined the essentials of the Feuerstein emphasis on modifiability with the developmental, play-based elements of DIRFloortime. After introducing these two discrete yet compatible models, there are chapters on islets of normalcy, the first an introduction to the concept, the second a guide for identifying them. The term "islets of normalcy" is pivotal in distinguishing the Feuerstein paradigm, which focuses on eliciting the strengths of the child with autistic-like (autistiform) symptoms rather than on documenting pathology. Following are a close reading of the most recent castings of the formal criteria for autism, and a call to strengthen the prevalence of the use of the term autistiform. Liberally illustrated with case examples, the theoretical section concludes with a discussion of how the needed paradigm shift from a quantitatively symptom-focused to a qualitatively strength-focused perspective has the potential to strengthen assessment of and interventions for children who present with autistiform symptoms.

This book is not a compendium of the latest fascinating neurological, biochemical or genetic research as it pertains to autism. Nor does it survey the most prominent treatment techniques. I have written this book, based on years of clinical experience, in the spirit of sharing: thoughts about the field of autism, reflections about the way autism is currently diagnosed, concerns about the misuse and over-diagnosis of the term autism, encouraging examples of children thought to be autistic whose lives were changed when we uncovered the child behind the symptoms; insights into how what might even be called an iconoclastic vision of autism can lead to dramatic progress beyond initial expectations.

A word about the term "autistic" itself as used in this introductory chapter and following is in order. For the most part in the field, the diagnosis of autism is used as a sacrosanct truism—a definable entity, the symptoms of which, like a disease, can be quantified readily and clearly identified. As the children in this book and their stories hopefully exemplify, such is not at all the case. I have found that the term "autism," as it appears commonly in the field, in actuality is being used to describe children who suffer from a vast range of communication difficulties, from extreme shyness to psychotic conditions and just about everything in between. It is not at all clear to me how research studies which purport to use autistic children as subjects can be certain that they have in fact studied autistic children, with the current diagnostic criteria of autism so elastic and with the use of the term so liberal.

So when I use "autistic" or "autism" in this introduction and throughout the book, I am using it as a reference point to indicate children who are/were thought to be autistic—although they might not be genuinely autistic at all, given the vast range of developmental challenges that the term "spectrum" allows. In the case vignettes I refer often to children who were "thought to be autistic," "diagnosed as autistic," "considered autistic" in order to imply a healthy doubt as to whether their original diagnoses were accurate. I have also used these kinds of descriptive phrases within the case stories in order to distinguish the formal diagnosis and the attendant presumptions that accompanied each child's referral information, from the more qualitative, functional and often deeper understanding of the child's difficulties and strengths which were elicited from our play-based dynamic, interactive assessments. Increasingly in the writing of these case stories, I came to use the term "autistiform," not to define the child but to describe the quality of the symptoms. This term is not a diagnosis. It is, in fact, an excellent descriptor in its *non-specificity*, and it means essentially "kind of looks autistic" or "sort of reminds me of autism." The reader may be shocked at this assumption: how can such a non-specific term enlighten the practitioner or aid the parent?

As I will argue in the chapter devoted to a close reading of the formal diagnostic criteria for autism, I observed that the current formal criteria for autistic spectrum do not offer the practitioner a clear, differential diagnosis, one which distinguishes between genuine autism as per Leo Kanner's (1943) original criteria—emotional cutoffness and an obsessive insistence on sameness engendering perseverative behaviors—and myriad potential false positives.[9] The diagnosis of "autistic spectrum," like the now obsolete diagnosis of Pervasive Developmental Disorder (PDD) in common coinage before the term "spectrum," is non-specific. A close reading of the current diagnostic criteria for "autistic spectrum," greatly expanded from Kanner's original criteria and with a corresponding loss of clinical specificity, reveals that the term "spectrum" barely provides the practitioner with enough information to conclude that the child's functioning "sort of looks like autism." In a later chapter, I respond to the implicit question: so why replace one general term, "spectrum," with another, "autistiform"?

The parents of most of the children presented in this book arrived at the Institute seeking an alternative type of assessment which they hoped would clarify the accuracy of the formal diagnosis they had received elsewhere. With nearly every case story in this book I have attempted to demonstrate how the children's progress ultimately revealed that the formal autism diagnostic criteria had led essentially to a misdiagnosis which had masked or even overlooked the underlying difficulties—and the positive potential—within each child. It is against this theoretical backdrop that each child's progress, sometimes remarkable, sometimes adequate, sometimes minimal yet still significant, is presented.

The story of each child in this book exemplifies in a different way and from a slightly different perspective how the layers of assumptions associated with a formal autism diagnosis were peeled away to reveal the child behind the autistiform symptoms. Jack's story tells of a delightful little boy, misdiagnosed in my estimation, and the struggle of his parents to overcome the burden of doubt a formal diagnosis engenders. The story of baby Sasha challenges the presumed need for early diagnosis and argues instead that *early understanding* of developmental needs and *early intervention* rather than *early classifying* serve the practitioner and the child more effectively. Annie visited the Institute only a few times, yet her anxious parents trusted that our formulation of Annie's considerable developmental problems—and her latent potential—would somehow lead to her much improved functioning. Davie's parents too wrestled with doubts, as they struggled to believe in his emerging potential. The story of Joe relays the challenges and the developmental changes that occurred when working with a middle-teenaged youth with entrenched symptoms and behavior patterns. Mikey's depressed mother had stopped talking to her child. Max had been misdiagnosed due to misinterpretations of his nonspeaking behavior. Josh is now a talented, normally functioning, productive adult, but as a preschooler he presented with what was far from a positive prognosis.

At the Institute, my colleagues and I assessed and followed the progress of likely thousands more children. The reader will note in these case stories that there was and is no set timeline for staff involvement with families who come to the Institute. During my tenure, there were families who came once or twice for an initial assessment or for a second professional opinion regarding their child's challenges and abilities. Often these few initial play-based assessments, which also employed DIR strategies that proved so compatible with the Feuerstein philosophy of modifiability, were nevertheless fruitful, in the sense that within a session or two there were positive, even if small, changes observed or elicited in the child's presentation. As we sometimes learned from the parents who phoned to update us years later, these small changes, along with the specific advice and recommendations we provided the parents, often had prompted a positive, creative change in the parents' approach and the treatment decisions they made for their child. The children whose stories are told here were seen at the Institute for varying lengths of time, ranging from only one or two assessment sessions, to intermittent follow-ups, to more frequent contact over a period of years.

In compiling these stories, I endeavored to select children for whom I had access to my personal notes, although in some cases I relied on my memories of dramatic, pivotal moments in the assessment or treatment of the children. In the instances for which I relied on memory, certain details, such as the exact play material or play-based learning activity I used to engage a given child, may not be accurate. However, the overall trajectories of developmental change, the direction and degree of progress, as described for each child, are accurate. Clearly, all names and identifying background details have been altered in order to protect the confidentiality of the children and their parents.

The case stories I selected pivot around my experience with the children in my office during assessment, treatment and follow-up sessions. I have focused on what transpired before my eyes within the confines of my office because that is what I could report accurately regarding the initial assessment of the children, my comprehension of their underlying difficulties, and the sometimes painful yet hopeful process their parents underwent during our consultations. Most of the children whose stories comprise this casebook were not able to enjoy the benefits of the multidisciplinary team of the Institute's intensive treatment program, which was created years later. However, the voices and the talents of my colleagues, from whom I learned so much, resonate through these pages as well.

Inspired by the Professor, the Institute's clinical staff aspired to make a significant difference in the lives of any and all special needs children. When families did not return, there was always a sense of sadness among the staff and an air of self-criticism: What had I missed? What more could have been done? My colleagues and I hoped to make a difference in the developmental trajectory even of a child with complex difficulties who visited us short term.

How I would have loved to compile a book comprised solely of astounding successes, one in which every child who arrived at the Institute previously diagnosed as autistic had begun, with our influence, to speak fluently, to learn at a normative level and to play happily with friends. That, of course, was not the reality of our work. However, it can safely and honestly be stated that, inspired and mentored by the Professor, my colleagues and I made a huge difference in the lives of hundreds of children originally thought to be autistic. We were able to meaningfully change children's prognoses and to disprove many clinical assumptions embedded in the reports of those who had evaluated the children elsewhere. It would not be inaccurate to say that as a team we were able to save many lives.

It is my hope that the case stories in this book will help strengthen parents struggling to trust their own intuition and belief in their child's capacities, regardless of the technical accuracy of an autism diagnosis. I hope that cumulatively these stories will help broaden and deepen the perspective of students of psychology and education so that they will enter into practice with a flexible and creative outlook regarding the autism diagnosis, rather than a rigid, constraining, deterministic or even fatalistic outlook. I also hope that in some way these stories will encourage instructors in the fields of psychology, counseling and education to expose their students to alternative ways of arriving at creative and reflective practice with children presumed to be autistic. While, yes, there are children who are genuinely autistic, as per a stringent interpretation of Kanner's original succinct formulation, and it is likely that their numbers are indeed increasing, nevertheless, an alternative model for the assessment and treatment of autism, as it can hopefully be taught and practiced, might just help stem the tide of falsely positive and misleading autism spectrum diagnoses flooding the field today. For those children for whom a misdiagnosis of autism has masked or obscured other developmental difficulties, and perhaps masked latent potential as well, I hope that this case-based description of an exciting, creative and satisfying way of working clinically will help reveal to many parents and practitioners the children behind the symptoms.

Notes

1 Reuven Feuerstein, Yaakov Rand, and Mildred B. Hoffman, *Dynamic Assessment of Retarded Performers: The Learning Potential Assessment Device, Theory, Instruments and Technique* (Baltimore, MD: University Park Press, 1979). The word "potential" was later changed to "propensity."

2 Reuven Feuerstein et al., *Instrumental Enrichment* (Baltimore, MD: University Park Press, 1980).

3 Dorothy R. Howie, *Thinking about the Teaching of Thinking: The Feuerstein Approach* (London: Routledge, 2003).

4 Alex Kozulin et al., "Cognitive Modifiability of Children with Developmental Disabilities: A Multicenter Study Using Feuerstein's Instrumental Enrichment-Basic Program," *Research in Developmental Disabilities* 31 (March–April 2010): 551–59.

5 Daniel D. Kurylo et al., "Remediation of Perceptual Organization in Schizophrenia," *Cognitive Neuropsychiatry* 23, no. 5 (2018): 267–83.

6 Stanley I. Greenspan and Serena Wieder, *The Child with Special Needs* (Reading, MA: Addison-Wesley, 1998).

7 Stanley I. Greenspan and Serena Wieder, *Engaging Autism: Using the Floortime Approach to Help Children Relate, Communicate and Think* (Boston, MA: DaCapo Press, 2009).

8 DIR is a registered trademark of the ICDL, the Interdisciplinary Council on Developmental and Learning Disorders.

9 Leo Kanner, "Autistic Disturbances of Affective Contact," *Nervous Child* 2 (1943): 217–50. Throughout this book, whenever the term "genuine autism" appears, I am intending a stringent interpretation of Kanner's two primary criteria, emotional cutoffness and an obsessive insistence on sameness, along with his secondary criterion of impairments in communication.

References

Feuerstein, Reuven, Yaakov Rand, and Mildred B. Hoffman. *Dynamic Assessment of Retarded Performers: The Learning Potential Assessment Device.* Baltimore: University Park Press, 1979.

Feuerstein, Reuven, Yaakov Rand, Mildred B. Hoffman, and Ronald Miller. *Instrumental Enrichment.* Baltimore, MD: University Park Press, 1980.

Greenspan, Stanley I. and Serena Wieder. *The Child with Special Needs.* Reading, MA: Addison-Wesley, 1998.

Greenspan, Stanley I. and Serena Wieder. *Engaging Autism: Using the Floortime Approach to Help Children Relate, Communicate and Think.* Boston, MA: DaCapo Press, 2009.

Howie, Dorothy R. *Thinking about the Teaching of Thinking: The Feuerstein Approach.* London: Routledge, 2003.

Kanner, Leo. "Autistic Disturbances of Affective Contact." *Nervous Child* 2 (1943): 217–50.

Kozulin, Alex, Jo LeBeer, Antonia Madella-Noja, Francisco Gonzalez, Naama Rosenthal, Ingrid Jeffrey, and Meni Koslowsky. "Cognitive Modifiability of Children with Developmental Disabilities: A Multicenter Study Using Feuerstein's Instrumental Enrichment-Basic Program." *Research in Developmental Disabilities* 31, no. 2 (2010): 551–59.

Kurylo, Daniel D., Richard Waxman, Steven M. Silverstein, Batya Weinstein, Jacob Kader, and Ioannis Michalopoulous. "Remediation of Perceptual Organization in Schizophrenia." *Cognitive Neuropsychiatry* 23, no. 5 (2018): 267–83.

Part I
Children

1 Jack
Misdiagnosis and the Burden of Doubt

That first entrance of Jack to my office is unforgettable. Just five, Jack was dressed in the creamy-white outfit of a karate aficionado. His karate garb was loaded with pockets, and they were bulging with treasures. His entrance was confident, full of energy and anticipation. His eye contact was direct, warm and engaging. There were no signs of fear or hesitation as he made that first connection with me. Because Jack presented with such a strong and open presence, it was clear that I could begin as with any typically developing child: "Jack, you've got pockets, and I see that they're full. What do you have in them?"

Jack's response was instantaneous. There was no need for me to clarify my query with a gesture such as pointing. Jack understood and responded immediately. Reaching into his pockets, he began to pull out his treasures. Transformers! Small plastic figures that, with a few twists and bends here and there, can be transformed from humanoid into monster, robot or vehicle forms. Jack promptly began to tell me their names and a little about the personality and role of each one. He pulled another one out of his pocket to frighten me, and laughed with delight when I feigned fear.

Within the first few moments of contact with Jack a number of key developmental points were clear:

- Jack communicated a strong presence and sense of self.
- He was open and warm.
- His fascination with transformers reflected normative, active, little boy play interests.
- He was at ease in the world of symbolic play, which requires a developmental sense of self and other (the non-self).
- He possessed the ability to enjoy and develop imaginative play worlds.
- He was responsive to personal contact and engaged readily in verbal communication, even with me, a stranger.
- He had a sense of humor.

What a delightful child! Whatever could be the developmental issue that had impelled his parents to bring him to the Institute?

His parents, meanwhile, looked distressed, sad and confused. Our conversation unfolded in English as much as possible rather than Hebrew, so as not to speak openly about Jack as he played in the room. His parents, it emerged, were in total shock, and they were mildly depressed as well. Barely a week before their visit to the Institute, they had taken Jack to be assessed by a well-known developmental specialist at a leading Israeli hospital. They had done so because there were aspects of Jack's verbal development that had been weak since he first began to speak. In preschool his social communication had been a cause for concern.

For several years now, Jack's parents had invested time and energy in dealing with these problems, and in fact, had decided to schedule an appointment with that particular specialist at the hospital because they were quite confident that Jack would be pronounced a normal, typically developing child. They were looking forward to a confirmation that their efforts of providing Jack with speech therapy had paid off and that Jack would emerge from the conventional assessment with a clean bill of developmental health.

They were stunned when the hospital's assessment team diagnosed Jack as autistic. I looked over the report of the hospital staff. Had they actually seen the same child I was seeing today? The difference between the hospital staff's and my perceptions of this child was immense—and frightening.

I tried to get a sense from his parents of the hospital assessment process. The hospital's developmental assessment team had arrived at the autism diagnosis using the criteria of the then in effect Fourth Edition of the *Diagnostic and Statistical Manual of Mental Disorders (DSM-IV-TR)*.[1] As will be discussed in depth (Chapter 13) within the *DSM-IV-TR*, like the subsequent *Diagnostic and Statistical Manual of Mental Disorders (DSM-5)*,[2] the criteria for Autistic Disorder were very broadly delineated. For example, in that former version any child who evidenced difficulty in initiating social conversations could garner a point toward an autism diagnosis.

I asked Jack's parents whether any of the specialists had played with him. "No." Had they attempted to engage Jack using humor? "No." At any time, were there several therapists in the room conducting a joint observation? "Yes."

In detective fashion, I tried to unravel why and how such a delightful, active, engaging child could find himself so seriously misdiagnosed by a team of experts. The tone of the hospital report was dry and clinical. It appeared that one assessing clinician had launched into a series of tasks with Jack without first attempting to create rapport and connection. Perhaps intimidated by this "cold start," Jack had spoken in single-word utterances, had repeated some words in echolalic (echoing) fashion, had evidenced a limited vocabulary, had used short sentences and had even started to stutter. When the tasks became too challenging, Jack's ability to concentrate had declined, and he eventually refused to continue.

His parents confirmed my impression from the report. The assessing specialists had not attempted to first engage Jack by using play and humor before launching into the various developmental tasks. The lack of genuine outreach to the child and the lack of any attempt to create rapport and thus reduce the child's anxiety had skewed Jack's functional responses away from the norm. The clinicians' ensuing impressions, and ultimately the diagnosis, leaned toward pathology: "Autistic Disorder, High Functioning."

Had the hospital assessment team actually played with Jack? This is an important question. In an assessment situation of a child with a suspected developmental problem in the direction of autism, it is critical that the assessor reach out to the child actively and energetically, using play materials, playful activities and most definitely humor, when possible, in order to engage and bring out the latent relational and interactional capacities of the child. The realm of play is where a child lives. Symbolic play offers an invaluable window into the inner world of the child, his or her interests, likes, dislikes, fears, the understanding of self versus other, the capacity for identification and imagination, and much more. Checking off a list of social communication dysfunctions without attempting to actively engage a communication-challenged child in interaction is comparable to the dentist working on a patient whose mouth is firmly shut!

For younger children or for those children who have not yet reached the level of symbolic play interest, which Jack clearly had, the assessor needs to get on the floor and attempt more sensory, physical types of interaction (with the parent in the room). This might include gently tickling the child's tummy or toes, rocking the child backward and forward, up and down as he or she faces you, or gently helping the child "jump" as assessor and child face the mirror. Simple activities like these, some derived from DIRfloortime strategies, unlock tension and enable the assessor to get a glimpse of the real child behind the symptomatic mask of emotional neutrality, fear and imploded communicative abilities. Fortunately, Jack's developmental level was well beyond that of a need for sensory play. He was already comfortable with imaginative, symbolic play.

If the hospital assessment team had not reached out playfully to Jack in order to reduce his anxieties and engage him, then it would appear that they had not encountered the real Jack. Rather, I began to assume, they had seen an intimidated child who had quickly intuited that these grownups were overly serious people. And if, as can often happen in developmental assessments, there were sessions with Jack in which a number of different therapists observed the child together, it would be easy to understand the intimidating impact on a child who suffers even the mildest social communication difficulty. The child might then present as inhibited at best and developmentally impaired at worst. Add to this the hyperelasticity of the formal autism diagnostic criteria, and one can see how readily misdiagnoses of the earlier classifications of Pervasive Developmental Disorder (PDD) and Autistic Disorder (AD) or the current Autistic Spectrum Disorder (ASD) occur. Jack was evidently a casualty of such a misdiagnosis.

A detailed developmental history of a child is indispensible in elucidating our understanding of a child's challenges in language, communication and relational development. For example, Jack's parents recalled the delayed onset of his spoken language, a period in which his eye contact became markedly poorer, and his reliance on gibberish at the time. Babbling and gibberish, when babbling starts to approximate words, are the basis for language development in a baby but, if noted in later developmental stages, are often considered signs of developmental problems. All too frequently such a constellation of developmental weaknesses such as Jack had evidenced in early childhood are, unfortunately, presumed to be early precursors, even confirmations of sorts, of the autism-related diagnosis the child may receive in later childhood. Such precursors can indeed signal serious developmental derailment or impairment. But not always, and certainly not with every child. In fact, in a child with a serious delay or impairment in expressive language, the onset of babbling and gibberish is wonderful, welcome news of rudimentary language acquisition.

It is so important that the developmental history not remain simply a history. The key questions the clinician must ask and the critical information the clinician must at least attempt to seek in the detailed history should help unravel the possible causative roots of a functional problem. Had there been a medical or an emotional trauma? No, but the parents' referral forms to the Institute noted that Jack had suffered from chronic ear infections and fluids. This is a developmental detail that, in my estimation, literally screams from the pages. An infant, toddler or young child who suffers from chronic ear infections and fluids would, by definition, have difficulty hearing. Language would sound garbled and unclear. Young children learn language by imitation, but if a child cannot hear accurately, his or her early attempts at language production will be compromised. Language development may be delayed. The child may feel discouraged and may somewhat withdraw, believing that adults around are not responding to his or her attempts to speak. Such a child is not necessarily at risk of being autistic, but that child will be at great risk of being misdiagnosed as autistic.

Too often the referral information we received for young children diagnosed or misdiagnosed as PDD, AD or ASD cited "chronic ear infections in infancy." In ironic fashion, I often told parents that this is "good news," helping us to unravel the developmental chain of events that frequently have lead in other quarters to a misdiagnosis of autism. The importance of this "small" developmental detail is often overlooked. Such was the case with Jack. The recent report from the hospital assessment team did not even mention his earlier problem with chronic ear fluids.

It appeared that other developmental factors had been overlooked or underappreciated in Jack's evaluation at the hospital barely a week earlier. For example, Jack had, in fact, undergone minor surgery for ear grommets, which had reduced the impact of chronic ear fluids. Subsequently, his expressive language had improved dramatically. The fact that Jack's eye contact had diminished for a time in babyhood was a concern. On the other hand—and this was good news—his parents had reported that, for reasons unknown to them, the situation had righted itself. Jack's eye contact had returned to normal expectations several years ago. Certainly on entry into my office, his direct, eager gaze was a delight. There was other worrying news, followed by good news, in the social realm. In his early preschool days, Jack had experienced difficulties making social contact. Now in kindergarten, he had friends with whom he enjoyed playing. Jack had changed.

The fact that a child's developmental difficulties have improved, beyond signaling that the child might have received the temporary assistance he required (such as Jack's ear grommet surgery), above all highlights to the clinician a simple and all-too-often overlooked fact: "This child is capable of positive developmental change."

In the early minutes of contact, I observed Jack and interacted with him playfully, but I had not yet begun to assess him in a more structured way. After observing and enjoying his warm and engaging manner, my intention was to interact with him at educational table tasks which would require perceptual focus, concentration and verbal capacities in comprehension and expression, and in the use of both concrete and conceptual language. I had already observed some of his developmental and personality strengths, as noted above. I considered these strengths important islets of normalcy, a key Feuerstein concept (elaborated in Chapter 10).

I was not worried about Jack. His energetic abilities were evident. I was much more worried about Jack's parents, to whom the hospital report had delivered a terrible blow to their belief in their own perceptions, intuitions, feelings and sense of parental competence. They were emotionally drowning in doubt. Preceding that recent process of conventional assessment, they had believed in their child. They had understood that his expressive vocabulary and syntax needed strengthening, and that he had been shy in his preschool. But they had invested time, energy and expense to strengthen him in these areas, and they were seeing progress. They had delighted in their son.

Their world collapsed, however, when Jack received the diagnosis of autism from the hospital assessment team, whose report was signed by a specialist in the field. Doubt is an insidious destructive force. Within barely a few days of having received the hospital report, Jack's parents were now racked with deep doubts about Jack, his abilities and his potential. "How could we have been so wrong? Our son is autistic. We have the report to prove it." Beyond this, and perhaps even more deleterious, they had been shaken to the core and were now doubting their own perceptions of and belief in their son. I saw that Jack's parents required attention to counter their despair, and I made a mental note to return to them after working with Jack on some cognitive (thinking/learning) tasks.

I had enjoyed the initial playful connection with Jack and his transformers, and he sensed this. There was an initial sense of rapport, to the degree that I felt the timing was right to suggest to him that we sit at the table and do some activities together. We warmed up with a few puzzles and matching tasks. The activities I chose were taken from a variety of cognitive materials that are part of the Institute's own battery of instruments for the qualitative, intentionally interactive assessment of young learners known as the Basic Learning Potential Assessment Device (LPAD-B),[3] a younger age-adapted version of the materials used with older learners, the LPAD.

Within the assessment framework developed by Feuerstein, interaction with the person being assessed is not only permitted, it is encouraged, unlike conventional assessment processes which often literally forbid the assessor's interacting with or assisting the learner in any way. Dynamic assessment materials do not have norms, and some are not even scored. Rather, the intricacies of the evolving learning process are qualitatively described. The assessor seeks a description of the *process* of learning. Rather than seeking a score of observed performance, the dynamic assessor aims to discern the impact of assessor-child interaction (mediation) on cognitive change. A child may begin a dynamic assessment task at a low level of processing and competence. But with the input of the assessor who interacts, mediates, verbalizes concepts, focuses the child and helps the child develop problem-solving strategies, by the end of a session the child may well be functioning at a much higher level of competence. Which is the true result? In the purview of the Feuerstein philosophy, the fact that the child has demonstrated the ability to change and to learn as a result of mediated interaction is a far truer reflection of the child's abilities than the initial performance, which may have been compromised by lack of confidence and/or lack of problem solving strategies.

To dynamically, qualitatively assess children with suspected autism in this unique unconventional way, the assessor retains this same mindset: "I am looking for a process of change within the child." The assessor seeks evidence of changes that run the entire developmental gamut from poor verbal expression to somewhat or even markedly improved verbal expression, from poor auditory attention to improved auditory attention, from poor eye contact to improved eye contact, from lack of pleasure in interpersonal contact to even brief evidence of delight in contact, to competence in relating, communicating and learning. To tally the symptoms of a child's initial presentation is *not* the end and aim of dynamic assessment. In the world of dynamic assessment of children thought to be autistic, the early symptom presentation is merely a baseline, a starting point for creative, interactive work geared toward coaxing evidence of change from the child, even microscopic changes. Symptoms are not the conclusive evidence of developmental impairment, and they do not tell the whole story of a child's developmental presentation. What is most critical is to discern, and invite, the child's latent strengths, those precious islets of normalcy referred to earlier. It is the child's latent strengths that can potentially enable the child to overcome, in part or wholly, suspected developmental pathology.

And so with Jack. We sat down at my little table and tackled some play-based cognitive activities that required, for example, selecting from several pictured alternatives the missing piece of a larger picture, creating picture sequences to form a logical short story or determining from several options the correct pictures associated with a target picture.

Jack had presented as strong in terms of his warm and energetic person-ality, as well as his emotional presence. In working with Jack, however, it soon became clear that he was less confident in expressing himself verbally. Often he knew an answer from the perceptual realm or could arrange pictures in a logical series, but he lacked the rich conceptual vocabulary and developed syntax (sentence structure) that could enable him to communicate his answers. He clearly comprehended most of the material. Yet it took him extra time to process the verbal mediation I offered him in order to help him to clarify his thinking process. These few cognitive tasks and our time spent at the table indicated that, indeed, Jack had some challenges in the area of verbal pro-cessing and in using richly expressive language.

However, it was also clear that Jack was not autistic. As we worked together at the table, he remained engaged, interactive and responsive. There was a sense of comradery and even warm humor between us. Working with him was an enjoyable reciprocal process. Jack's presentation was far from being gen-uinely autistic, as posited in 1943 by Leo Kanner.[4] Jack was not cut off emotionally nor was he suffering from obsessively perseverative (repetitive) behaviors. Jack, as I have observed, was a charming little boy, with some difficulties in language processing and with an attendant lack of confidence in tackling verbally-based tasks.

Aware of the enormous shortcomings of the autism diagnosis, and its too-easily attained clinical non-specificity (the criteria having expanded ex-ponentially since Kanner's succinct formulation), I did not even consider using the word "autistic" to summarize Jack's challenges. He possessed con-siderable, even charismatic, personality strengths on which to draw in order to improve in his weaker areas, given a little extra help from a warm and capable speech therapist.

It was clear to me that Jack needed to remain among other typical chil-dren for an additional year in a regular kindergarten, rather than be placed in a special educational setting (as is common in Israel for children con-sidered to have special needs) in which he would find himself among speech- and language-impaired children. With continued educational integration (inclusion) Jack would enjoy sustained immersion in a milieu of capable, social and verbally expressive children, a milieu that would clearly continue to strengthen him.

Basing their recommendations on their foregone conclusion and diagnosis that Jack suffered from autism, in all its diagnostic non-specificity, the hospital team had recommended that Jack be transferred in the coming school year to a small special kindergarten and be placed among children suffering from a variety of expressive language impairments, including autism. For Jack, nothing could have been worse. While he might have received sixty minutes of speech therapy per week within that special kindergarten, he would have paid a heavy developmental price, given the lower level of the play and social communication skills of the peers among whom he would have been immersed daily.

It was necessary now to return the focus to his parents, who had sat sadly and silently as I worked with Jack at the table. The terrible power of doubt, and the terrible power of a diagnosis to hijack a parent's own belief and delight in their child! So discouraged were they about their son that Jack's parents, it appeared, had not noticed or internalized the lively, attentive interaction he displayed as he sat with me at the table, happily engaged in age-appropriate kindergarten level learning tasks.

Jack's parents had been so burdened by their doubts and worries about him that they had missed the wonderful, warm quality of his interactions in my office. Focusing more on his weaknesses, they had not seen the improvements that had occurred in his conceptual language use during our work together. Identifying a child's weaknesses and working with them is very different from identifying a child *with* his weaknesses and thereby allowing the diagnosis or clinical label to function as a determinant of the child's abilities and, in a sense, the child's very identity. The newly received autism diagnosis had not elucidated Jack's situation. For his parents, the diagnosis was instead now functioning like blinders.

I gave Jack some play props to use with his transformers and, letting him play on his own, moved over to my desk to sit opposite his parents. Their questions to me showed that the burden of doubt about Jack weighed heavily on their feelings and thoughts about him: "Don't you think Jack should be transferred to a special kindergarten? Why not? Don't you agree that he is autistic?"

One of Professor Feuerstein's ironclad principles was that he was always prepared to make himself available to see any child who came to the Institute, when the child and parents were accompanied by the Institute staff person who had begun the dynamic assessment process. Often, however, this meant that the child along with the parents might have to wait outside his office for a long time. I took a chance, evaded his secretary, and phoned the Professor directly. Jack's educational path and his future were at stake. The Professor's vast clinical experience, broad knowledge and deep wisdom could be invaluable in reducing the doubts that clouded these parents' very relationship with their child.

"Professor Feuerstein, there's a child in my office who has been diagnosed as autistic. I feel that this is totally inaccurate. His parents are now tormented by doubts as to whether to place him in a special kindergarten or keep him in a regular kindergarten." The Professor's response: "Bring the child and his parents to my office immediately."

On entry to Feuerstein's office, Jack immediately dug into his pockets to show the Professor his many transformers. The Professor feigned fear, and Jack laughed with delight. After a few more minutes of interaction as well as some further warmly interactive cognitive work at his huge desk, the Professor announced to the parents: "Your child has nothing to do with autism. The autism diagnosis is absolutely inappropriate for Jack. It is critical that your child remain within a regular educational setting, among talkative, expressive, playful children. Your child is not suffering from PDD or autism. He is a casualty of 'MMM.'" "MMM" was Feuerstein's own in-house ironic term for "Man-Made Madness." While never one to ignore a child's specific difficulties, he knew full well the pitfalls of certain diagnoses which, rather than elucidating a child's developmental functioning, only served in their over-generalization to essentially create a "disorder."[5]

Feuerstein was a man of remarkable intelligence, clinical knowledge, wisdom, intuition and insight. He had accumulated more than sixty years of clinical experience since the end of World War II. Further, he possessed a warm, deep, charismatic personality, and he spoke with a sense of conviction. This was exactly what Jack's parents needed. The strength of Feuerstein's insights about their son helped push them beyond the shadow of doubt. They left his office having decided to let Jack repeat a year in a regular kindergarten setting. We set up a follow-up appointment. With the scales tipped toward Jack's remaining in a regular educational setting, I looked forward to following his progress.

The initial two meetings with Jack took place within a month's time. We scheduled a third dynamic assessment meeting, to take place a few weeks later. I assumed, wrongly as it emerged, that those first two appointments had made a dramatic positive impact on the parents. They had arrived in the depths of despair, believing that the conventional diagnosis they had received from the hospital was accurate and that their son was autistic. However, rather than seeing Jack's earlier preschool difficulties or his current mild language weaknesses as confirmations of developmental pathology, the Professor and I had reaffirmed Jack's overall positive developmental path, highlighted the hearing difficulties that might have impeded early language development, observed in session his impressive interactional and personality strengths that could enable him to overcome residual weaknesses, and had reached a positive prognosis, given Jack's continued educational inclusion.

Unexpectedly and inexplicably, Jack's parents dropped off the radar for the next six months. They phoned to cancel that third appointment. In a later outreach phone call to them, the situation became clearer. They wanted to embrace our recommendation that Jack repeat a year of regular kindergarten—but. They were still buffeted by waves of doubts and fears: "What if the learning and social demands of a regular kindergarten prove too much for Jack? What if educational inclusion leads to his feeling frustrated and a sense of failure? What if Jack really is autistic?" Perhaps, they agonized, he really needed a small, attuned special education environment where he would receive several hours of speech and occupational therapy each week, even if he had to be placed among special needs children, all of whom suffered from social communication and expressive language impairments.

In fact, before his arrival at the Institute, Jack had already spent a year in a special needs preschool because an earlier evaluation at age three had concluded that he was "developmentally delayed." During that year, by parental report, Jack had benefitted from the small, attuned special education preschool. His expressive communication abilities had improved. The evidence of that early childhood progress was still echoing during his two visits to the Institute. Jack now presented as a warm, interactive typical child with only minor language processing weaknesses. The special setting had done its job for Jack. However, we had concluded that now it was time for Jack to move on. He possessed considerable personality strengths of warmth, humor and imaginative play skills that would serve him well among other typically developing children. His developmental history had virtually proven that Jack possessed the capacity to grow and change significantly. We were confident that his language-processing skills would blossom with his continued educational inclusion.

Before receiving the hospital's assessment that had concluded that Jack suffered from Autistic Disorder, his parents had decided that his regular kindergarten setting suited Jack well. As already noted, they had expected the hospital's assessment to be a rousing confirmation of all their hard work. We completely concurred with the parents' original estimations of their son's progress and his strengths. However, the hospital's formal assessment of Jack, as I have relayed, had cast that shadow of doubt on their own convictions about their son. The power of a diagnosis, and not the power of Jack's expressed and latent strengths, was poised to determine Jack's future. I have seen it all too often.

My follow-up phone call to his parents was a long one, in which I attempted to strengthen the parents in their own original and correct understanding of their child's abilities. I added that my colleagues and I had coached and supported many parents to maximize the benefits of inclusion within the regular educational stream, and that our Institute team would be happy to help support Jack's continued educational inclusion. At the end of the conversation, the parents' direction was still not clear. Jack's mother, in particular, still sounded perplexed and fearful for his future.

Several months later, Jack's parents phoned to report that after much deliberation, they had decided to continue to integrate Jack in a regular kindergarten. Jack was doing extremely well there. They reported that he had made "huge progress." He was doing well socially. He had some good friends. Although Jack's teacher had observed that he had mild difficulty with word retrieval and that he had problems describing a story sequence, he was doing well in learning the basics of reading and writing. Despite this encouraging news, doubt and fear about his abilities and his future were still perceptible in the parents' tone. Nevertheless, they set up another appointment for him, during which I noted Jack's continued good progress. Following this latter appointment, Jack did not return to the Institute. The parents' phone updates or requests for advice became increasingly less frequent and then ceased.

I never forgot Jack. Impulsively, several years later I made a follow-up phone call to Jack's parents. During that call it became clear that Jack and they had come a long way. Jack was now functioning well with some supports in his regular third-grade classroom. Although certain aspects of the learning program were challenging for him, he was holding his own. Socially, he was doing extremely well, enjoying warm friendships and participating in various activities with peers.

Gratifyingly, in response to Jack's positive progress, Jack's parents too had changed. They were no longer plagued by doubts about Jack's ability to grow and change. They were enjoying Jack. They loved his charming personality and appreciated his successes as he continued to make progress in overcoming the communication challenges, but not autism, that he had suffered in early childhood.

Notes

1 American Psychiatric Association, *Diagnostic and Statistical Manual of Mental Disorders: DSM IV-TR* (Arlington, VA: American Psychiatric Association, 2000).
2 American Psychiatric Association, *Diagnostic and Statistical Manual of Mental Disorders: DSM -5* (Arlington, VA: American Psychiatric Association, 2013).
3 Rafael S. Feuerstein, Reuven Feuerstein, and Louis Falik, *Learning Potential Assessment Device-Basic: Examiner's Manual* (Jerusalem: ICELP, 2009).
4 Leo Kanner, "Autistic Disturbances of Affective Contact," *Nervous Child* 2 (1943): 217–50.
5 Louis H. Falik, *Changing Destinies: The Extraordinary Life and Times of Prof. Reuven Feuerstein* (Bloomington, IN: Xlibris, 2019), 217.

References

American Psychiatric Association. *Diagnostic and Statistical Manual of Mental Disorders: DSM IV-TR*. Arlington, VA: American Psychiatric Association, 2000.
American Psychiatric Association. *Diagnostic and Statistical Manual of Mental Disorders: DSM -5*. Arlington, VA: American Psychiatric Association, 2013.
Falik, Louis H. *Changing Destinies: The Extraordinary Life and Times of Prof. Reuven Feuerstein*. Bloomington, IN: Xlibris, 2019.
Feuerstein, Rafael S., Reuven Feuerstein, and Louis Falik. *Learning Potential Assessment Device-Basic: Examiner's Manual*. Jerusalem: ICELP, 2009.
Kanner, Leo. "Autistic Disturbances of Affective Contact." *Nervous Child* 2 (1943): 217–50.

2 Sasha

The Specter of Early Diagnosis

Baby Sasha looked lost as he sat silently on the carpet in my office. He gazed at the few toddler toys I had placed beside him and touched them absently. Although he manipulated them now and then, he was not playing with them. He was not investing his actions with affect (emotion) or meaning. He did not look up with interest, curiosity or even the apprehension which would be expected from a child, not yet even a toddler, who found himself in a strange setting. He did not appear anxious and so he did not move closer to his parents for comfort or reassurance. In fact, Sasha did not express any feelings. Rather he sat gazing with an intense focus (hyperfocus) at the play objects before him. He did not engage in any exploratory play that expressed curiosity, wonder or pleasure. He looked so lost, alone and forlorn.

At the age of eighteen months, Sasha appeared distant from a warm emotional connection with his parents, from playful involvement with objects and from the energetic exploration of his surroundings, as would be expected from an almost toddler. He appeared detached and, in his detachment, appeared to suit well the central criterion for autism of extreme emotional cutoffness, long ago determined by Kanner. In many professional settings using conventional means of assessment, Sasha's detached and nonresponsive presentation would likely have quickly garnered him an autistic diagnosis of some kind.

However, on the encouraging side of the ledger, I noticed that there was one critical criterion for autism that was completely lacking in Sasha's presentation: there was no sign of any perseverative (repetitive) behavior, no hand-flapping, body-rocking, circuit-walking or shaking/spinning of objects. Very often autism assessment reports I had read from professionals who had used conventional autism assessment protocols had noted a child's silent withdrawal, for varying reasons, but appeared to have overlooked the fact that the child lacked any perseverative behaviors. This should be a strong signal to professionals that genuine autism, as per a stringent reading of Kanner's criteria, may not be a fact. Other developmental forces could be at work. The absence of any perseverative behaviors in Sasha's seriously aloof and non-communicative profile of behaviors was significant. If an essential element of the original Kanner-based autism diagnosis was missing, I considered this highly encouraging. Rather than perceiving Sasha as autistic, I sensed that this little child, behind his symptoms, was developmentally stuck. In a different way, so were his parents.

In a kind of contrapuntal response to Sasha's quiet detachment, Sasha's parents were suffering intensely from a crippling combination of anxiety and discouragement. Sasha's mother looked and sounded depressed. She spoke openly about her fears for Sasha's present and his future, and of her sense of both hopelessness and helplessness in the face of her little boy's problems. Sasha was the youngest of her five children, so this mother had much experience in parenting. However, she had never encountered a developmental glitch. Recently she had quit her job in order to spend more time at home with little Sasha. Clearly overwhelmed and frightened, she appeared more burdened and depressed than her husband, although he too was clearly suffering.

Despite her palpable discouragement, Sasha's mother did say that at home Sasha at times "seemed" to understand what was being said to him; sometimes he even responded to simple requests. But he was not yet speaking at all. He had not begun to use gestures to communicate. He did not wave goodbye, or clap his hands in excitement. Instead of gesturing for help, Sasha simply cried.

As of this, our first meeting, Sasha had not yet been formally diagnosed as belonging either to the category of autism or to the then extant PDD. However, the specter of the word "autism" was foremost in his parents' minds, weighing them down with a sense of fear. Indeed, on the basis of the first minutes of this initial observation of Sasha, I would have expected these parents' first consultation with specialists using conventional assessment procedures for autism to yield that formal diagnosis.

Sasha thus far had been able to evade early diagnosis. He had enjoyed the good fortune to be treated privately by a talented, highly regarded speech therapist who had assessed him functionally, that is, descriptively. She had not referred to a listing of symptoms in order to arrive at a diagnostic category. Comprehending Sasha's need for reciprocity, for the give-and-take of eye contact, vocalization, imitative sounds and words, she had been providing him with intensive treatment using DIRFloortime principles twice weekly for a few months now. The modest signs of progress that the parents could report were in large part due to her efforts.

Before getting down on the carpet to play with Sasha, I spent at least forty-five minutes in intense discussion with his parents, sensing their need for emotional first aid. My goal was to attempt to ease them away from their sense of hopelessness, to create even a modest degree of openness in them toward a new way of thinking about their child's developmental predicament. In their frustration and despair, these parents had already "self-diagnosed" their child. I wanted to help them begin to experience a paradigm shift away from a diagnosis-focused mode of perception and intervention toward Feuerstein's functionally descriptive way of working, in which every glimmer of the child's positive presence and rudimentary communication is considered significant, a tiny islet of the ability of the child to change within the sea of developmental challenges. Sasha's parents desperately needed to be exposed to a different theoretical perspective and to receive practical tools of playful, interactive communication so that they could experience a sense of hope, access their energy and begin to move forward.

I explained to Sasha's parents the pitfalls of the overly elastic formal diagnostic criteria for autism with their attendant risk of false positives, pointing out that this elasticity leads to a near arbitrariness of an autism diagnosis that is tragically treated in some professional quarters as an irrevocably negative developmental sentence. Not so! It was also important to introduce them to the Feuerstein notion of "islets of normalcy" (Chapters 10 and 12), so that his parents could begin to identify even microscopically small evidence of potential in Sasha. Above all, I stressed what was possible, based on my clinical experience: that with the right intervention, including the parents' own energetic playful involvement and emotional outreach to him, Sasha's situation could yet prove to be highly modifiable.

The Specter of Early Diagnosis?

Before continuing Sasha's story, it is important to respond to an implicit question. Some readers might find the title of this chapter perplexing: the *specter* of early diagnosis? Isn't it most important to ascertain the correct clinical label at the earliest possible developmental age? After all, most developmental and mental health care professionals feel that they have not done their job if the assessment does not yield a formal diagnosis of a child's problem, with the symptoms carefully identified and tallied. Certainly, it *is* important to identify, acknowledge, and understand, as early as possible, the developmental realms which are weak or impaired in a child, in order to help the child as soon and as effectively as possible. And it is important to clarify through medical testing whether observed soft signs of compounding developmental problems are rooted in genetic, metabolic or neurological influences which might require medical intervention. But within the paradigm in which I worked for nearly twenty-five years, more cogent than a diagnosis was the need to functionally understand the child's symptoms, to identify the child's latent strengths and to create facts on the ground regarding the modifiability of the child's symptoms and the child's latent strengths.

A child's strengths or the modifiability of symptoms are not ordinarily reflected in a conventional autism diagnosis. Further, the diagnosis runs the risk of defining the child according to his or her difficulties. Like a frequently referred to example from the field of medicine, "Nurse, please attend to the tonsillectomy in the next room," it is too easy to conclude that the diagnosis summarizes the child's being with a sense of finality. Feuerstein taught that there is another way of viewing the autism diagnosis: with great caution.

From the Feuerstein perspective, autism is a potentially modifiable state and not a fixed trait.[1] Young children are capable of meaningful change—to the extent that the autistic label need not necessarily apply to the child in a few years' time. However, if an autism diagnosis limits our perceptions and our thinking about an individual child to generalized preconceptions about autism, the preconceptions associated with that diagnosis can do enormous damage to individual young children, overlooking their strengths and their unique latent potential for developmental change, and prematurely foreclosing certain treatment options or goals as "unrealistic."

In my work over a generation, I encountered hundreds of young children who had been diagnosed conventionally in other settings as autistic. By the time some of them arrived at the Institute, their autistic diagnosis was no longer applicable, with the child perhaps requiring some supplemental therapies or other focused interventions to strengthen them in the normative developmental path that I perceived was possible for them. There were other children, a much smaller percentage than the numbers usually reported, for whom the autism diagnosis was accurate and offered clarity. For these children and for the children whose symptoms were severe, entrenched and perhaps complicated by genetic or neurological difficulties, here too, the intent of our assessment was not to label the child but to seek strengths and evidence of modifiability, and to actively probe how to improve the child's presenting profile. For the vast majority of children whom my colleagues and I assessed and treated, an early autism diagnosis had obscured the underlying influences of the child's developmental difficulties and/or, more worryingly, had focused treatment intervention on autism as the problem, rather than addressing underlying issues such as anxiety, trauma, hearing problems, sensory difficulties, emotional factors and so on. These underlying factors can turn out to be *root causes*, or at least strong influences, of a child's developmental difficulties, often treatable and highly modifiable when recognized as such, with the signs of what at first appear to be autism fading and even disappearing as the child improves.

It is widely assumed that an early diagnosis of Autism, Autistic Spectrum Disorder, or the former Asperger's Syndrome and Pervasive Developmental Disorder, fulfills that purpose of identifying, acknowledging and understanding developmental impairments related to communication difficulties. But such a conclusion—that a diagnostic label advances our *understanding* of a child—is inadequate.

Years ago, at a major international conference organized by Stanley Greenspan and Serena Wieder on the treatment of autism, Professor Feuerstein presented a paper titled insightfully, "Early Detection: Blessing or Curse?" In this treatise, later published as a monograph,[2] he pointed out the many pitfalls related to the early diagnosis of autism. Using a term like the "pitfalls" or the "specter" of an early diagnosis may seem shocking and even outrageous if one is committed to arriving at a diagnostic label, on the assumption that a diagnosis can be equated to clinical understanding. However, if a conventional diagnostic process is laden with less-than-convincing logic and generalized assumptions, as questioned throughout this book, then the diagnosis will not lead to deeper clinical understanding and clarity. The conventional diagnostic process will lead instead to a misconception of the child's actual difficulties and a diagnostic label that is little more than an approximate overgeneralization.

A diagnosis in the field of medicine is an extremely useful and life-saving concept. I have sometimes reflected that psychology, my chosen field, seems to suffer from an inferiority complex in relation to the field of medicine, in which high-powered medical technology and biochemical analyses provide numerical results at a powerful degree of resolution and accuracy. Certainly, the field of psychology never ceases to strive for assessment measures that can provide numerical results with the highest degree of test validity and reliability. However, in cases of suspected autism, it is critical to move beyond the scores, the numbers and even the norms, and to create a dynamic descriptive profile of the child's strengths (islets of normalcy), as well as a descriptive assessment of the modifiability of the child's symptoms and the types of energetic, playful interaction which have been shown during the assessment to be effective in weakening these symptoms. A dynamic, playful, interactive assessment strives to yield what Feuerstein called a "profile of modifiability" and a prototype of strategies for further positive work.

An early diagnosis of autism, from the Feuerstein perspective, potentially offers more risks than clarity. However, early *intervention*, which is attuned to the unique, functional needs of the child who appears autistic and which seeks to amplify the child's strengths and latent potential, is essential. Although shadowed by their worries that Sasha was autistic, Sasha's parents had decided to bypass any formal diagnostic process. Instead, they focused their energies on early intervention rather than early diagnosis, seeking positive, effective play-based assistance for him using DIRFloortime.

Sasha's Story Unfolds

While observing Sasha sitting silently on the floor, I attempted to give his parents some initial information about the paradigm in which we worked in order to help release them from the grip of their fears and frustration. It was eminently clear that Sasha was in a perilous developmental situation: not talking or even babbling, not playing, not gesturing, seldom making eye contact—it was just a matter of time until he would be formally diagnosed as autistic and recommended for placement, as is common in Israel, in a special education setting where although he would receive speech and other therapies, he would ironically find himself in a social/educational milieu among solely nonspeaking youngsters. Regardless of how talented his therapists might be, in such a special setting what peers could Sasha model and with whom could he practice playing and communicating?

Now it was time to get down on the floor and attempt to play with Sasha, to try to create what DIR proponents refer to as "circles of communication" and what Feuerstein termed "reciprocity." The scope and intensity of Sasha's developmental symptoms were clear. But where was the child behind the symptoms? Might it be possible through playful interaction to find, perhaps even to create, some islets of normalcy in the deep sea of developmental symptoms before me? Might it be possible to ignite in him a few tiny sparks of emotion, humor, interest, warmth, connection or curiosity?

On the floor with Sasha, I attempted a range of baby playtime activities and made a few interesting and heartening discoveries. As noted earlier, Sasha was visually hyperfocused on the toys in front of him. Was he really not interested in emotional connection or did he simply prefer taking in information through the visual channel? Could the visual channel be used to create the missing link to emotional connection? I picked up a small glittery toy fish on a string which fascinated him visually and held it between our faces, waving it back and forth. Sasha made intermittent eye contact. His eye contact was not warm, but it was not indifferent. Rather, it was gentle and sensitive, and it communicated: "I'm in here, but I'm stuck."

Bearing in mind DIR principles of paying attention to a range of sensory modalities, I gently touched his toes and waited to see if he would signal me with some eye contact that he wanted a little more gentle touch. Sasha looked up! I did not speak at this point but touched his toes again to signal that I had received his visual, nonverbal message. A tiny circle of communication was created. Reciprocity.

From the tactile to the visual modality: I detached the mirror from the wall and set it in front of us on the floor. Using this indirect and less threatening form of eye contact, we sat on the floor, with Sasha in front of me. With the mirror facing us, Sasha's gaze toward me was clearly steadier, a small but encouraging point.

Later, away from the mirror, I made a few more playful overtures, blowing bubbles toward but not at him. Sasha watched them float. Then I began to sing to him softly. Was I imagining it, or at the end of our session did Sasha seem less tense and forlorn? I thought so. Embedded in these simple play maneuvers, I had observed a few islets of normalcy and he had closed a few tiny circles of communication—some eye contact, perhaps a flash of interest in the bubbles, decreased tension in his body. There was no sign of a smile yet, nor any sign of pleasure in interaction.

Later I reflected that in applying play-based Floortime strategies for increasing his eye contact, it had not been terribly difficult to get that eye contact. It was not hard work. That detail alone was significant, shedding light on the fact that, although Sasha's overall developmental profile appeared to be serious and complex, the few symptoms I challenged using play had not been intransigent. The little boy behind the symptoms was in there—stuck, lonely, but perhaps not all that far away.

There is a difference between a symptom constellation in which the symptoms are ironclad and stubbornly entrenched and a symptom constellation in which the very same symptoms are light and more readily malleable. By using some of the conventional autism symptom checklists or *DSM* criteria, two children with the same symptoms, though in varying degrees, may arrive at the same "score" and yet be worlds apart in terms of prognosis.

A child with less entrenched symptoms, and who is temperamentally and sensorily more accessible, will respond and improve with less intensive investment. Yet even the child with more entrenched and stubborn symptoms may well still prove highly modifiable. He or she will require a greater investment of intensive energy to be enticed, warmly and playfully, into contact and relationship. Sasha's symptoms at first glance appeared daunting and convincing, but tiny cracks in his shell of aloneness had appeared.

Nevertheless, Sasha needed help. That was clear. Fortunately, the brief play-based foray with him on the carpet, and his minimal but nevertheless perceptible responses, suggested to me that he would respond positively to a massive infusion of the interactive play strategies of DIR, which his speech therapist was already using.

In the clinic of the Feuerstein Institute, the mandate of the multi-disciplinary staff was primarily to provide interactive qualitative dynamic assessments of children's functioning and to provide recommendations that could help each child realize the perceived but still latent potential. In later years, the Institute opened a program for intensive treatment. However, when Sasha arrived, this program did not yet exist. Sasha needed intensive "play work" immediately.

I attempted to arm his parents with a number of recommendations that I had found were usually feasible for even emotionally overwhelmed parents to carry out. Based on years of experience inspired by the guidance of Feuerstein, I knew that these mini-interventions on the part of the parent can gradually catalyze a maximal effect. The metaphor I often used to coax depressed, depleted and discouraged parents to try to reach out to their nonresponsive child more proactively was an unusual one. "Have you ever tossed a pebble into a pond?" I would ask parents. "Do you remember how that little pebble can make much larger waves? Well, the guidelines I am giving you can function in that way. The little changes you make, in initiating contact with your child and in responding to him, have the potential to make waves and to stimulate significant developmental progress down the road."

I proceeded to explain to Sasha's parents the Feuerstein technique of soliloquy.[3] Simplifying the explanation and keeping it as practical and doable as possible, I encouraged his parents to speak generously, amply with Sasha, using a rich vocabulary. About what? About what is happening, both around him and within him (feelings); about what has happened and about what is going to happen. I tried to fortify them against discouragement if Sasha did not respond, citing that research in conjunction with the Institute had strongly linked soliloquy techniques to improved language output.[4] At the same time, I advised them to speak slowly and clearly, so that Sasha, whom I assumed was listening even if he were not responding, would not have to expend energy and effort in discerning sounds; this would leave him more energy for potentially expressive responses.

Contrary to the recommendation common in Israel that Sasha should immediately enter a special education setting where, it is widely thought, "he would get all the therapies he needs," I urged his parents to continue to maintain Sasha in a regular educational setting among speaking toddlers. In a special setting, I emphasized, Sasha might receive excellent therapies, but he would miss completely the social milieu of normative peer models of speech, play and social interaction. In a typical toddler setting, he would enjoy a rich verbal, functional and social milieu to which he could ultimately connect. Sasha's parents intended to continue to provide him with speech therapy, privately, with the talented speech therapist who was already working with him using DIR techniques.

I coached Sasha's parents about the critical role of imitation in learning in general, and in language development in particular, and explained to them how important it is to create imitative interest and abilities even if the child appears unable or uninterested in doing so. This is done by sensitizing parents to be on the lookout for opportunities for imitation: "If your child makes the slightest sound, even involuntary cooing, sighing, sneezing or coughing, position yourself so that you have the child's eye contact and imitate the child's sounds. If he continues with another sound, that is wonderful news. Keep going and continue to imitate, creating from inadvertent sounds a nascent conversation or, in DIR phraseology, 'circles of communication.'"

Sasha was not even gesturing—for example, pointing. Consistent with Feuerstein's approach, which takes into account the ability of the brain to learn from repeated action, I advised Sasha's parents to create gestures which did not yet exist—waving goodbye, clapping with excitement, pointing—by physically holding his hands and helping him perform these functions in context.

Since Sasha had responded positively to play in front of the mirror, I suggested that his parents do daily "mirror time" with Sasha, holding him on their lap in front of the mirror, while singing, cooing, making faces and above all being sensitive to the quality and duration of the eye contact they are encouraging. Mirror time, of course, is a wonderful opportunity for building imitative interest and skills, with the adult imitating the child's conscious or even inadvertent babbling, gibberish, words and songs as well as hand, lip, mouth and facial movements.

At home Sasha was often plunked in front of videos for far too many hours. Sasha's lack of interpersonal initiative was thereby being reinforced, much to his detriment. I explained to his parents that this lonely, isolated, all-absorbing activity did not serve his urgent needs for contact, relationship and shared activity, and advised them to limit his screen viewing to no more than thirty minutes a day. Finally, I suggested to his parents that they generously increase his DIR treatment hours, since both Sasha and they would require, at least in the short term, a concentrated, intensive input of developmental and supportive energy. I looked forward to seeing Sasha again in about one month's time.

Three months later, at the age of one year and nine months, Sasha and his parents returned for a follow-up consultation. His parents had decided not to place Sasha among special needs youngsters, but to maintain him in his same small nursery setting among typical children. They had increased the number of weekly DIR sessions with his speech therapist from two to three times a week.

Sasha's mother spoke first, giving a discouraging litany of her worries: still no gestures, no behavioral response to instructions and no social interaction in his nursery setting. In fact, Sasha's mother seemed more tense and worried than during our first meeting. At the same time, paradoxically, the parents concurred that there was much good news. Sasha had begun carrying out play tasks that involved construction and early puzzle-making skills at a level advanced for his age. More encouraging still was the fact that there was progress in terms of relationship and communication. They were seeing signs of Sasha's sense of humor. Sasha had begun approaching his parents for warmth and occasional cuddles. He had started to play in toddler fashion near his siblings and, at times, actually with his siblings.

Sasha had begun to speak! Sasha had acquired three words: "teddy," "ball," and "doll." He had also begun to repeat "many words" that he heard. In addition to his first words, the evidence of newfound interest in imitation was wonderful news and an exciting prognostic sign that Sasha was opening up to the world and beginning to master one of early childhood's most critical skills—the imitation of speech and language. Despite their lurking apprehension about his future, Sasha's parents were noticing Sasha's much delayed and still rudimentary but undeniable progress.

On the face of it, nothing dramatic had happened to bring about these encouraging changes. The parents had simply been attempting to apply our recommendations. Yet the little changes his parents had attempted were indeed making waves. Although they had not opted for maximum, intensive Floortime which would have given Sasha—and themselves—more opportunities for creating and closing circles of communication, they had wisely increased the frequency of the speech therapist's intervention and had maintained him in a nursery setting among typical peers. Both of these factors would surely impact positively on Sasha's incipient language development. Despite their fears and the aura of discouragement surrounding them, they had attempted as best and as often as they could to speak generously to Sasha, without demanding any response, and to respond vocally or verbally to any of Sasha's sounds and, lately, to his words.

I have learned that it is always a good sign when developmental progress occurs concurrently in more than one developmental realm. For example, if a child's eye contact improves, that is positive and significant news. However, if a child's eye contact, his smile response and his interest in rolling a ball to a parent improve concurrently, that is wonderful developmental news. The child's whole proclivity toward contact, relationship and communication is then beginning to shift. Such was the case with Sasha, and yet his parents seemed unable to delight in this news.

In contrast to his initial visit, it was clear that Sasha was beginning to respond. Still overwhelmed with worry about the developmental impasse that had challenged Sasha only a few months ago, his parents understandably could not really relax and feel confident about his future. I decided to enlist the deep insight and charismatic intervention of Professor Feuerstein, whose ability to discern islets of normalcy in a child was more than matched by his gift for reaching parents. With the power of his sixty years of extensive clinical experience and his warm, deep personality, he was so often able to help parents see the child behind the symptoms.

I picked up the phone to Feuerstein's secretary, and we soon found ourselves in the Professor's office. Neither he nor Sasha disappointed. Soon Sasha was babbling richly as the Professor imitated him. Responding to the Professor's warmth, Sasha appeared alert, alive, warm, relaxed and more reciprocal than I had observed during that first session in my office. In Feuerstein's office, Sasha even emitted a two-word approximation. Many fears were dispelled as the parents watched their son open up and respond so dramatically. Sasha's parents left that day strengthened and encouraged. I reiterated to his parents the basic recommendations they had received in our first visit, and I assumed that I would be seeing Sasha soon for other follow-up consultations.

Months passed and Sasha's parents did not return. I phoned them to inquire about his progress. The news was good. Sasha was now being seen by two DIR-trained therapists. Sasha was also continuing in day care among typical toddlers. Sounding much more relaxed and happy, Sasha's father reported that "Sasha continues to improve all the time."

Although I saw him only twice, and that during a period of great uncertainty in his life as he made those first hard-won steps toward healthier functioning, I never forgot little Sasha. In a way which I cannot fully explain, I felt certain, even in those initial appointments, that Sasha possessed normative abilities, and perhaps beyond normative. I had to wait a long time to hear what had happened to little Sasha.

When Sasha was three years and three months old, his parents phoned my office. They wanted to bring Sasha to the Institute and show me with pride and pleasure just how far Sasha had come. No longer a toddler struggling to close developmental gaps, Sasha, now nearly a preschooler, entered my office with a real sense of presence, ready to engage in some interesting age-appropriate play-based learning tasks. Sasha had been successfully toilet trained. On his head, consistent with his parents' religious background, Sasha wore a yarmulke. That he was willing to keep the yarmulke on his head was in itself significant, since often children with special sensitivities will not agree to wear head coverings of any sort.

We sat down together at the little table. A color-matching puzzle was far too easy for Sasha. He spontaneously named the animals as he fit the corresponding pieces into the wooden puzzle form. When I asked him questions about the animals, such as "show me the one that likes to swim in water," I noticed that there was a slight hesitation on the level of input (receptive language). It took Sasha a little extra time to process a question, and a little more time to formulate the language needed to respond (expressive language). There was nothing developmentally pathological about his need for a little more time to process language. Sasha simply needed people to speak to him slowly and to give him patient, supportive time for language processing before he responded.

When we turned to preschool-level story books, Sasha shone. He listened raptly as I read to him in Hebrew the popular children's books *Good Night, Gorilla*[5] and *Where's Spot?*[6] His visual hyperfocus, which at the age of eighteen months might have been enough to clinch a PDD or an autism diagnosis in some settings, was now serving him well. Sasha was exhibiting excellent attention and comprehension, listening to and observing every detail of the story. After listening to each of these books, Sasha decided to retell each one. He did this beautifully, turning the pages, describing with emotional coloration the development of each story and even letting his sense of humor shine through.

At this stage, there was little to add to the armory of recommendations I had given his parents in the past. Sasha had truly crossed the critical threshold from being at risk for developmental pathology. He had advanced to normative and even above-normative functioning. "We know," said his parents. "We are so proud of him, and we wanted you to see how wonderfully he is doing."

Only two years before, Sasha's parents had been wrestling with the specter of an early autism diagnosis, a possibility that had deeply concerned them even though Sasha had not been formally diagnosed as such. In Israel, an early diagnosis would have led to Sasha's early entry into the special education system, where he would have encountered capable therapists but no normative peer milieu to pull him along. Sasha's parents had opted for early intervention using developmentally attuned DIRFloortime, by a speech therapist who had guided Sasha toward reciprocal communication. Sasha's parents' few visits to the Institute had served to support and to consolidate the direction they had already chosen. Sasha had done the rest.

Notes

1 Rafael S. Feuerstein, ed., *Feuerstein on Autism* (Jerusalem: Feuerstein Institute, 2019).
2 Reuven Feuerstein and Louis H. Falik, "Early Detection: Blessing or Curse," in *Enhancing Cognitive Functions: Applications across Contexts,* eds. Oon-Seng Tan and Alice Seok-Hoon Seng (Singapore: McGraw-Hill, 2005), 147–88.
3 Reuven Feuerstein et al., *A Think-Aloud and Talk-Aloud Approach to Building Language: Overcoming Disability, Delay, and Deficiency* (New York: Teachers College Press, 2013).
4 Ibid.
5 Peggy Rathmann, *Good Night, Gorilla* (New York: Puffin, 1994).
6 Eric Hill, *Where's Spot?* (New York: Puffin, 1980).

References

Feuerstein, Rafael S., ed. *Feuerstein on Autism*. Jerusalem: Feuerstein Institute, 2019.

Feuerstein, Reuven and Louis H. Falik. "Early Detection: Blessing or Curse." In *Enhancing Cognitive Functions: Applications across Contexts*, edited by Oon-Seng Tan and Alice Seok-Hoon Seng, 147–88. Singapore: McGraw-Hill, 2005.

Feuerstein, Reuven, Louis H. Falik, Rafael S. Feuerstein, and Krisztina Bohacs. *A Think-Aloud and Talk-Aloud Approach to Building Language: Overcoming Disability, Delay, and Deficiency*. New York: Teachers College Press, 2013.

Hill, Eric. *Where's Spot?* New York: Puffin, 1980.

Rathmann, Peggy. *Good Night, Gorilla*. New York: Puffin, 1994.

3 Annie

Emergence from the Shadows

When pale, dark-eyed Annie, aged two-and-a-half, walked into my office with her parents, it was easy to see at first glance why and how she had been diagnosed by staff at a prominent health clinic as suffering from Autistic Disorder (AD), at the time the common diagnostic reference before the addition of the term "Spectrum," for any child who was considered autistic. But my attention was drawn in equal measure to her parents.

The atmosphere in my office that day was heavy with the parents' grief and concern about their daughter, who had been diagnosed six months earlier. Annie's mother appeared to be functioning under a cloud of depression. She clearly was demoralized, and experiencing deep-seated doubts about her ability to effectively help her child. She expressed fundamental doubt, as a result of the AD diagnosis, as to whether Annie could improve. Impelled by intense anxiety, Annie's father could not stop asking me questions. In a tone as gentle and supportive as possible, I tried to quiet the parents' initial waves of distress, communicating to them, "Often the diagnosis is not the whole story when it comes to child development. Please try to relax. Let me observe Annie and then attempt to play with her. We will talk later."

At first I quietly regarded Annie as she wandered about the room. Annie was indeed a concern. She presented as a child in serious developmental trouble. Annie did not make eye contact with me, or with her parents for that matter. Poor eye contact of itself need not necessarily be a feature that clinches a child's diagnosis of autism, although, sadly, it is often mistakenly used as one of the diagnostic "clinchers." What are important to distinguish, rather, are the variations of the child's eye contact. Even an initially shy but typically developing child may avoid eye contact, but as the relationship warms, the child's presentation can transform, perhaps within minutes, from avoidant to expressive to even warmer eye contact. Annie, however, appeared intensely committed to avoiding my gaze and that of her parents, as she moved around my small office, without any interest in exploring the toys. But the most compelling aspect of Annie's presentation was the shadow of sadness mingled with anxiety that haunted her dark eyes.

My office was equipped with a small table on which I often put out preselected toys that I sensed could engage a given child's temperament, interests and developmental level. There was also a mirror at child's eye level and a large, softly padded U-shaped object that can gently enfold a child who likes to rock on it or cuddle in it, wrapped in a blanket. When turned upside down, the U functioned as a little tunnel, for crawling or hiding under, for climbing and sliding on, or for pushing objects like cars through the opening.

Annie just continued to wander aimlessly around the office. She did not engage purposefully, meaningfully or expressively with any of the play objects. She did not smile nor did her behavior express any pleasure in movement or in a simple play activity, as might be expected with a typically developing child her age. Even slight vocal utterances can be a welcome key which the therapist can turn to advantage and use to open the door to developmental change. However, Annie uttered no words that day. In fact, she hardly emitted any vocal sounds.

In addition to her silence and her intensely avoidant eye contact, I noted with concern that Annie appeared emotionally remote. Her avoidance was tinged with more than reticence. Worryingly, her presentation reflected the essential "cutoffness" which Kanner in 1943 denoted as an essential feature of genuine autism. Annie's initial presentation suggested an autistic condition, and a rather serious one at that—or so it appeared at first glance. Yet, there were no stereotypical or perseverative (repetitive) behaviors—a significant clue that autism may not apply. Also, there was that dark shadow of apprehension, anxiety and sadness that I had noticed. That was my second clue as to her developmental state. A child who is anxious and sad is not totally cut off from or indifferent to his or her surroundings. Anxiety and sadness are emotional responses.

There were other complications, so to speak, in her profile and in her life. Her parents interchangeably spoke Hebrew and Spanish, their native tongue. So at home Annie had to process and ideally respond in two linguistic channels. In the past year, Annie's life had been graced with the addition of a baby brother, who was developing well and whom Annie assiduously ignored as effectively as she avoided emotional contact with her parents. Slight and pale, Annie was also suffering from severe eating problems, agreeing to ingest only baby formula and salty treats. Her appetite, like her communication profile, was tight and closed.

A more common and conventional assessment of Annie's developmental problems might have proceeded as follows. The physician, psychiatrist, psychologist or other practitioner might have begun by utilizing a checklist of behaviors and symptoms that can characterize autism. With these checklists, such as the Childhood Autism Rating Scale (CARS)[1] or the Autism Behavior Checklist (ABC),[2] the practitioner tallies symptoms, and in some cases the degree or frequency of each symptom, with the total score indicating whether the child is autistic or not (and if so to what degree). Increasingly, practitioners use the play-based modules of the Autism Diagnostic Observation Scale (ADOS)[3] which includes an in-depth parent interview[4] and which yields a scored result. However, more frequently encountered in my work in Israel was practitioners' use of the *Diagnostic and Statistical Manual of Mental Disorders (DSM,* versions *IV* and *5)*, the key diagnostic resource of the mental health field, with its comprehensive listing and description of symptoms that characterize a large range of developmental, emotional and psychiatric conditions.[5]

Autistiform (autistic-like) developmental symptoms, like the proverbial tip of the iceberg, can often be easy to spot: the child does not make eye contact, the child does not talk, the child does not play or engage emotionally, the child's behavior is perseverative and so on. In a conventional diagnostic process, the identification and subsequent tallying of symptoms is the goal. The key questions underlying conventional diagnosis are: What is wrong with the child? What are the child's symptoms? What name do we give this constellation of symptoms?

Throughout this casebook, I suggest that the questions we should be asking are: Who is the child behind the symptoms? How can we reach this child? How can we strengthen the real child so that the symptoms weaken and diminish while the inner core of strength and potential within the child begins to emerge?

Having observed the sobering and worrisome presentation of Annie for at least twenty minutes, I wanted to see whether, how and to what degree, even within the span of an initial appointment, it might be possible to effect some change in her challenging presentation. Based on observation, I understood why she had been diagnosed, correctly or incorrectly, as falling into the autistic category. Now, using interactive play strategies, I wanted to see how and to what degree her initial presentation might be modified. Was it possible to coax a little eye contact from her? Might it be possible to woo her into a flash of warmer, playful contact? Could a range of activities induce her to make sounds, which I could then imitate to create a sense of rudimentary conversation?

Clearly, it is important to know where a child is experiencing developmental difficulties. We *do* need to be able to identify areas of weaker functioning or outright dysfunction. However, beyond this identification of symptoms, we need to be able to understand what is happening within and to the child. It is commonly assumed that if we arrive at a diagnosis, then by definition we understand what is happening with a child. In my experience, nothing could be further from the truth.

Each of a child's tangible, visible symptoms is a world in itself. Like the shoots of a green plant, symptoms have intricate roots. They can have myriad reasons. These reasons may be physiological, genetic, developmental, emotional and/or psychodynamic, among others. The reasons and root causes may be significant, critical and illuminating but, within the Feuerstein philosophy of working dynamically, these reasons need not necessarily be determinants of a child's potential. For both parents and professionals, the interpretation and understanding of each symptom constellation, with particular attention to symptom gradation, intensity, modifiability, subtleties and nuances, is critical. Behavioral and functional manifestations of a developmental challenge like autism are not necessarily monolithic and unchangeable. They are in many cases transform-able. Were Annie's?

Just observing Annie's symptoms as she appeared frozen in her aloofness and anxiety would not lead her out of her developmental impasse. Drawing from the principles and strategies of DIRFloortime, I attempted to engage Annie by using a variety of play materials and activities: bubbles, rocking and gentle touch.

Following each attempt to "play" with her, I quietly backed off and gave Annie the space she seemed to want. A little dance of sorts was created. I moved closer to Annie, tried blowing bubbles, or tickling her or rocking her and then I backed off. She would tense at each "intrusion" into her physical and emotional space, but when I backed off after each attempt, Annie seemed calmer and less anxious. With each foray into Annie's space, I thought I detected a hint of better eye contact. Was it just my imagination or did Annie fleetingly look at me through the cloud of bubbles I blew silently?

Later, Annie was definitely interested in climbing on the upside-down U, or sitting astride it facing me and letting me rock her in it as I sought oppor-tunities for eye contact. Although her overall pattern of interaction was avoidant non-interaction, there were tiny but significant sparks: her glances at me, a tiny smile of pleasure as she rocked, and a sense, not observable but nevertheless palpable, that Annie was listening intently to my comments to her parents as I explained to them why I was playing with her in a certain way. On one hand, there were some encouraging signs of response during play with Annie, but on the other hand, these were only the tiniest sparks of connection or communication. How to coax these sparks into a flame of developmental energy?

A parallel metaphor for these little sparks of life is "islets of normalcy," that is, small even microscopic evidence of normative functioning, surfacing within an ocean of symptoms, a key concept appearing throughout these case stories. Professor Feuerstein breathed new life into the not unfamiliar concept of islet of normalcy, regarding it as an "anti-symptom," and using it with particular emphasis in relation to children thought to be autistic (elaborated in Chapters 10 and 12).

So in observing Annie, I was seeking more than proof of her only too evident developmental difficulties. Of course, it was necessary to note her specific difficulties in order to formulate a kind of descriptive baseline of her presenting functioning, but, since I was working in a dynamic model, I was accustomed to assuming that with the right kind of intervention, that baseline would prove modifiable.

After well over an hour of observation and rudimentary play interaction, Annie's few islets of normalcy comprised a short list:

- Fleeting eye contact with me as I blew bubbles.
- Interest, perhaps even pleasure, in climbing on and rocking in the large, soft U apparatus, with brief intermittent eye contact.

- A shift by the end of the session from an extremely tense presentation to the sense that Annie was more relaxed.
- Even the absence of any perseverative, stereotypical behavior such as body-rocking, spinning of objects or hand-flapping could be interpreted as a significant islet of normalcy in Annie's profile.

These islets were small, in fact microscopic, in proportion to Annie's overall detached presentation. They were also fleeting or of limited duration, and fragile; that is, they were not stably expressed in her presentation: "Now you see them, now you don't."

After my foray into play with Annie, as challenging and subtle as that proved to be, I was faced with a dilemma. I had seen miniscule islets of normalcy in a stormy sea of developmental dysfunction. As daunting as Annie's largely withdrawn and unresponsive presentation was, these islets were significant. Would they prove sufficient to begin to build a healthier developmental repertoire? The attempts at interactive play with Annie using both visual and kinesthetic (action/motion) play modalities (bubbles then rocking), with only faint glimmers of response, indicated that a considerable investment of interactive energy would be required in order to yield results. What could I offer these anxious and discouraged parents to help them assist their daughter effectively?

Several years later the Institute offered a program of intensive therapy. Children would attend once or twice weekly for a morning of various therapies provided by a multidisciplinary team. But this program did not exist in Annie's day. Besides, Annie's family lived far from Jerusalem, and a once-weekly intervention in her situation would have done little to move her along developmentally. Her situation was serious, and the need for effective, intensive intervention as well as for sustained support for her parents was extreme.

As I had promised the parents at the outset, at the end of the "play work" with Annie, I refocused my attention on them. The initial challenge was whether I could move the parents from their discouragement and anxiety toward a stance of gathering enough energy so they could help their daughter in a meaningful fashion. As with the parents of other children considered autistic whom I assessed, I began by providing the parents with basic information which could help move them toward a paradigm shift in the vision of their child—from hopelessly and terminally impaired as autistic to developmentally challenged perhaps, but essentially modifiable (the degree to be determined with hard work). Her parents also needed to understand the limitations of conventional assessment, focused as it is on symptom collection rather than on the expansion of islets of normalcy. They needed to understand as well the limitations of diagnostic labels, and the importance of appreciating those islets of normalcy.

Emotionally overwhelmed as they were, each of Annie's parents had adopted a style of interaction which did not serve her development. Mother's depressed feelings and lack of hope left her little energy for interacting with Annie.

So Annie's mother tended to withdraw from Annie emotionally. Annie's father, impelled by anxiety, adopted a style of interaction which I commonly observed in my work—quizzing the child or otherwise pressuring the child to speak. Intending only the best for his child while trying so hard to penetrate her rather convincing autistic-looking shell, the father pressured Annie to respond: "Say 'bubbles' Annie, 'buh-buh.'" At home he repeatedly tried to make Annie name the food she wanted before he gave it to her. The results only frustrated her father and drove Annie further inside herself. Because of his deep anxiety about Annie, he often spoke in her presence about her "autism" and her difficulties. Annie needed help, and her parents needed support and guidance.

The challenge was to somehow piece together the essential elements of a developmental rescue program for Annie, and for her parents, using a combination of resources and recommendations to be applied outside the Institute. I explained to Annie's parents how and why the approach at the Feuerstein Institute viewed an autistic condition as inherently modifiable and not inherently hopeless. They could not be expected to carry out recommendations for interacting with their child if they did not at some level internalize a sense of plausible hope, and feel as well that they had some concrete tools for interacting with their daughter who so effectively resisted interaction.

Perceiving that Annie's situation was modifiable but at the same time aware that Annie required more than the occasional follow-up appointments with me, during that session I phoned one of the leading DIR professionals in Israel and made the referral. She agreed to meet with the parents and to see Annie several times a week as well as to train the parents in the developmentally attuned and interactively beneficial play strategies of DIR which they could then incorporate into their daily interactions with Annie. The parents appeared enthusiastic about this opportunity.

Then there was the challenge of Annie's educational setting. Reviewing the referral information supplied by her parents, I noted that the professionals at the health clinic which had diagnosed Annie as autistic had strongly recommended that Annie enter a special preschool class, known as a "communication class," for autistic children within the educational system. While Annie would then have been surrounded by a team of highly qualified special education teachers and therapists who could offer her weekly speech and occupational therapy, she would have also been learning among eight other young children, all of whom would be suffering from serious communication deficits. With whom could she speak if and when she wanted to? From whom could she learn social and play skills? With whom could she simply have fun? And if the approach in this special class stressed behavioral training rather than warm relationship building, how could Annie internalize the basic sense of interpersonal reciprocity and pleasure in contact that she so desperately needed? The risk was too great that the benefits of the therapies she would receive in a communication class would be offset by a social environment deficient in inspiration and opportunities for peer interaction, communication and just plain fun.

Contrary to the recommendation that Annie enter a special communication class, I strongly recommended that Annie be integrated in a playgroup or in a small private preschool of typically developing children roughly a year younger than Annie. In this way, Annie, nearly three, would be integrated among talkative and playful two-year-olds. Fortunately, Annie was small for her age. Three-year-olds, already speaking and well-entrenched in their play skills, might also have been an option for her educational integration, but something in Annie's super-sensitive presentation suggested that she might fare better among younger and, therefore, perhaps less threatening children. Had she been placed among three-year-olds, Annie would likely have required an integration aide to help her interface with these more active and interactive youngsters. Since the Israeli educational system did not provide such aides for three-year-olds at the time, seeking and employing a skilled aide would have meant extra stress and considerable expense for these already overstressed parents. Integration among typical two-year-olds seemed the most appropriate and feasible option.

The combination of intensive DIR, guided by an expert and utilized daily with Annie at home, along with educational inclusion, offered the best chance for a more positive prognosis, and for Annie to emerge from her (nearly) convincing autistic presentation and begin to develop in a more typical direction. However, Annie's parents urgently needed what could be called "Communication Development First Aid Tools" to help them begin to replace their discouragement with practical ways to relate to her. The first recommendation was a strong caution to them *not* to speak of Annie's difficulties, her presumed autism or their worries about Annie in her presence. My assumption was that Annie was listening and absorbing their anxiety about her. Next, I urged her father to avoid quizzing Annie or in any other way pressuring her to speak. If Annie were to speak and engage with the world, she would need to be warmly wooed to speak, but not pressured to communicate.

My essential challenge with Annie's parents, as with so many parents whom I met over the years was, at the very least, to equip them with the knowledge before they left my office for the first time, that if they wished to have any hope of their child changing toward being a communicative being, they needed to begin by talking to their child. I attempted to help the parents understand why it was so important that they speak to Annie generously, with a rich vocabulary, using a normative tone of voice. I wanted them to address the Annie behind the symptoms, to communicate to her that they knew, or at least sensed, that she was in there. What this meant in practical terms was that they should not meet her silence with their own. For example, during daily activities, they needed to speak normally to Annie, describing what was happening within and around her, *without* any pressure for her to speak. At the same time, working from the assumption that Annie was capable of acquiring language, I urged them to speak slowly and clearly to her. As Annie became more attuned to the verbal language channel, she would comprehend better and hopefully begin to imitate what she heard, if the models of speech around her were slow and clear. I gave them concrete examples. Before going outside, for example, their speech might sound like: "I'm looking for your flowered boots right now. Oh, this one is hard to put on. Your sock is all bunched up. There, we got it. Good thing we got these on because it's raining really hard outside."

Why should a parent bother with such a monologue if a child is presenting as verbally unresponsive and uncommunicative? Because through such monologues, the child is exposed to the rhythm, prosody (musical cadence), vocabulary and syntax (structure) of language. More importantly, in addressing the child in this way, the parent is in essence addressing the child *behind* the symptoms. When the parent speaks to the child who appears to be unresponsive or even incapable of speech, the parent is actually communicating a belief that the child is indeed capable of communication. Feuerstein, as alluded to in other chapters, called these parental monologues "soliloquies." During my career at the Institute, I found that when parents engaged in such monologues even before the child exhibited any encouraging signs of readiness to speak, their soliloquies served as a critical catalyst for the child's later language and communication development.

As we talked in this first session, I could see that Annie's parents were wrestling with many conflicting thoughts and emotions: "Can there really be hope for our daughter? Will it make a difference if I talk to my silent child? Many other professionals are recommending a special setting. Annie is so far behind her age level developmentally. Is it realistic to consider integrating her among younger children, and typical ones at that?" At the end of this session, Annie's parents were still struggling with doubts and anxiety, but they appeared willing to give our recommendations a try.

Given Annie's challenging presentation, I assumed that her parents would return for frequent follow-up visits, perhaps once every four weeks, to get tips and guidance on how to capitalize on and accelerate her progress. Since it appeared that Annie would soon be starting an intensive DIR program nearer to home, we fixed our next follow-up appointment for a month later. Several weeks later Annie's father phoned to cancel that appointment. He then cancelled again shortly before the following scheduled appointment, although he continued to maintain some phone contact.

Subsequently, from the father's intervening phone calls, I tried to piece together a picture of Annie's progress. Her father had stopped pressuring Annie to speak or to perform; Annie appeared happier; she appeared to be enjoying herself more, and she even laughed sometimes. Her eye contact was improving, and she was starting to declaim words. Her father sensed that Annie understood more. Showing an encouraging sign of emotional responsiveness so unlike her initial detachedness, recently Annie had shouted "Yuck!" when her parents were arguing. Trying to keep the pulse of change alive via these phone calls, I continued to encourage the parents to speak to Annie generously "as if she understands everything." I reminded her father not to pressure her, and encouraged her mother to play with her in whatever way felt comfortable.

At last, roughly five months after her initial visit, Annie's parents returned for a much-delayed follow-up. There were a number of very encouraging changes. Above all, Annie did not appear as anxious or as emotionally remote and cut off. Her parents seconded this observation with their experiences at home. They reported that Annie was now more comfortable walking with them hand-in-hand. She had begun taking a parent's hand and directing it to whatever toy she wanted. She had started to point to objects, and she had begun quietly paging through picture books. They added that she even appeared to enjoy having a simple story read to her.

What had the parents done to help bring these changes about? Annie's parents had tried DIR with the specialist for only a few sessions. They could see the positive impact on the early stages of shared attention and pleasure in relating, but to my dismay, and for reasons unclear, they had discontinued her DIR sessions. However, they had stopped using Spanish at home and spoke to Annie in Hebrew only. They were trying to refrain from talking about Annie's difficulties in her presence. They were talking to her more (soliloquies) and they were making an effort not to pressure her to respond verbally.

In the office I observed some encouraging islets of normalcy with regard to speech and language development. Annie was now babbling a bit. Her mother was concerned that at night Annie lay in her bed and babbled gibberish. Was this normal? Was this all right? In fact, I explained, it was an excellent sign. Babbling and talking gibberish are normative phases of language development in which the infant or toddler experiments with sound production and baby's own language. They are necessary steps in the development of language. For Annie, this was occurring several years later than normal, but at least she was vocalizing, and occasionally letting slip a word or two. Her babbling or gibberish was a very good sign. I encouraged them to keep talking to her using a rich vocabulary and in normal fashion, using complete but shortened sentences. I reminded them to continue to speak about what is happening around her and within her—her feelings—but to remember to speak slowly and clearly, so she could absorb the communicative intent.

Her parents stated that they themselves did not feel emotionally ready to integrate Annie in a typical educational setting. They had decided to keep her at home for the summer and then to place her in a special education setting four months later. After mornings in the special setting, Annie's mother was considering integrating her in an afternoon playgroup for typically developing children.

Annie arrived for a third follow-up session roughly ten months after her first session—far from ideal timing for a child with such serious developmental challenges. Happily, there were remarkable changes. Annie even looked better. Her color was healthier, and her parents reported that her appetite had improved. Annie was far more open and relaxed. The weight of pressured anxiety that had typified her in that first session had largely dissipated. On the emotional/behavioral front, parental reports varied. On one hand, she seemed to be tolerating her little brother better. On the other hand, she occasionally had night fears. Sometimes she hit her mother. While the latter are not "desirable" behaviors, they did indicate responsiveness to the world and its emotional demands. I noted these changes as emerging islets of normalcy.

She had come a long way from her intense avoidance of ten months earlier. Developmentally, Annie had taken some very big steps. There were even signs of emergent symbolic play. In my office, Annie pretended to feed a baby doll. At home, Annie had begun to play with a soft plush rabbit. The ability to represent through pretend play is a significant indication of a developing sense of self and other, and it signaled for Annie an important developmental turning point.

Annie had begun to speak! Granted, at the age of three she was miles behind the expectations for her chronological age, but in comparison with where she had been ten months earlier, she was miles ahead. Her parents relayed that at home they could even have "conversations" with her as they spoke to her normally, while Annie responded in brief utterances of one to three words. There were even warm utterances that indicated an interest in relationship and a sense of humor. Recently Annie had looked at her mother and laughingly called her a "potato head!"

The parents were continuing to make every effort to apply some of the essential Golden Rules from DIR and Feuerstein intervention which I had shared with them—"respond verbally to her every effort to communicate" and "talk to her richly." They had wrestled with my recommendation that Annie be integrated, but ultimately they had opted to place her in a small special education preschool. There were six children in the class, three of whom did not speak and a fourth with only episodic words. Annie had moved from a nonverbal presentation, through babbling, to incipient speech (short utterances) within roughly ten months. I again suggested that if placed among typically developing children younger than her, Annie would likely enjoy a breakthrough in her speech development.

And then, to my dismay, Annie and her parents disappeared from the radar screen, apart from rare phone updates and brief phone consults. It would be a long time before I saw Annie again. Roughly eighteen months after her first visit, when Annie was four years old, her parents brought her back to the Institute—a changed child. Annie was talking, laughing, engaging and playing with enjoyment. I could detect shadows of her earlier, deeper, emotionally-based developmental disturbance—in her lack of confidence, in her language which should have been richer and more fluid, in the sense of fragility that still characterized her presentation. But overall, what a delight it was to see her at this level of functioning!

Her parents brought me up to date. Soon after their last visit when Annie was three years old, they had begun to feel dissatisfied with the lack of progress she was making in the special education communication class in which they had decided to place her. In midyear, they pulled her out of special education and integrated her within a typical preschool setting for three-year-olds. Annie's developmental pace then began to accelerate.

Annie's mother, who earlier had struggled so hard against feelings of discouragement when her daughter had been diagnosed as autistic, felt increasingly encouraged as Annie improved. Her mother now invested more time and energy in her relationship and activities with Annie. She had begun to enjoy reading to and playing with her daughter, with obvious benefits to Annie.

In response to her marked progress, Annie's father had begun to let go of his anxieties about her future. He had begun to enjoy her in the present, as a sweet, normal little girl. Although faint shadows of her past difficulties were still perceptible, Annie was no longer crippled by those difficulties. Once again, Annie and her parents dropped off the radar.

Then, four years after Annie's first visit to the Institute, I received a call from Annie's mother. Annie was now six, finishing her second year in a typical kindergarten. She was due to enter a typical first grade in the fall. Would I see Annie and provide a report on her readiness to continue in a regular educational setting?

The sweet, charming, warm, open and communicative child who entered my office a few weeks later bore no trace of the detached, imploded, silent, starving two-and-a-half-year-old of years ago. Since Annie presented as so responsive as she entered, I quickly decided to bypass play activities and to challenge her with a range of cognitive (learning) activities in order to get a sense of her readiness for a regular first grade class.

Beyond her technical reading readiness, Annie was enthusiastic about learning to read, and she demonstrated at least average abilities for entry into first grade. She did not shy away from challenges: she wrestled with questions that required her to process complex or abstract information and she gamely tackled arithmetic problems which were difficult for her. Throughout this "soft" assessment using cognitive activities, Annie remained involved, responsive and reciprocal.

Toward the end of our meeting, I wanted to get an impression of Annie's emotional understanding. Together we looked at some educational materials, photographs of children in various social situations experiencing a range of emotions. Annie was raptly interested, commenting on what the children were doing and what they were likely feeling.

Annie was interested in the photos, but could she relate with empathy and identify with the feelings she saw depicted? "What makes you happy, Annie?" I asked. Her response: "When I have friends." And later, "What makes you sad, Annie?" Annie: "When friends won't play with me." Annie had come a very long way. Although she might still require some afterschool help to support more advanced conceptual thinking and mathematical reasoning, she had the basic social interest and even the sophisticated air of a "with it" child, ready to take on new challenges.

Annie's parents too had travelled a long road. Her father no longer anxiously spoke of his "autistic" child but simply enjoyed his lively daughter.

Mother had undergone a dramatic transformation. She had come to believe in Annie's abilities, and in her own. Years ago, several specialists had classified Annie as autistic and, because they thought that autism was immutable, they could provide no toehold of hope or the kind of practical advice that would help Annie progress significantly.

When Annie's parents were supported to adopt an alternative interpretation of their daughter's difficulties and were equipped with some practical tools for relating to, communicating and playing with Annie, their belief in their daughter's ability to progress was strengthened. Feeling more confident in themselves and in Annie, they transferred her into an educationally inclusive setting. All these factors combined to create a situation in which real growth was possible for Annie. In a sense, not just Annie but her parents as well emerged from the shadows.

Notes

1 Eric Schopler et al., *Childhood Autism Rating Scale, Second Edition (CARS-2): For Diagnostic Screening and Classification of Autism* (Torrance, CA: Western Psychological Services, 2010).
2 David A. Krug, Joel R. Arick, and Patricia Almond, "Autism Behavior Checklist-ABC," in *ASIEP-3* (Torrance, CA: Western Psychological Services, 2008).
3 Catherine Lord et al., *Autism Diagnostic Observation Schedule (ADOS-2)* (Torrance, CA: Western Psychological Services, 2012).
4 Michael Rutter, Ann Le Couteur, and Catherine Lord, *Autism Diagnostic Interview-Revised* (Los Angeles, CA: Western Psychological Services, 2003).
5 *DSM* criteria pertaining to autism receive closer attention in Chapter 13.

References

Krug, David A., Joel R. Arick, and Patricia Almond. "Autism Behavior Checklist-ABC." In *ASIEP-3*. Torrance, CA: Western Psychological Services, 2008.
Lord, Catherine, Michael Rutter, Pamela C. Dilavore, Susan Risi, Katherine Gotham, and Somer L. Bishop. *Autism Diagnostic Observation Schedule (ADOS-2)*. Torrance, CA: Western Psychological Services, 2012.
Rutter, Michael, Ann Le Couteur, and Catherine Lord. *Autism Diagnostic Interview-Revised*. Los Angeles, CA: Western Psychological Services, 2003.
Schopler, Eric, Mary E. Van Bourgondian, Glenna J. Wellman, and Steven R. Lane. *Childhood Autism Rating Scale, Second Edition (CARS-2): For Diagnostic Screening and Classification of Autism*. Torrance, CA: Western Psychological Services, 2010.

4 Davie

A Longer Journey

The jury was still out for adorable Davie, three-and-a-half years old when he first arrived at the Institute. A few weeks earlier, Davie had been seen by several autism specialists in other professional settings. A well-known psychologist and a highly-regarded speech therapist were convinced that Davie's profile suited the *DSM-5* criteria for Autistic Spectrum Disorder (ASD). However, two other speech therapists had concluded that Davie was suffering from a delay in language acquisition with attendant social challenges.

The story of Davie is one of a longer, gradual and steady journey to achieve the normative potential that could be perceived even in his initial session. Genuinely shaken by the conflicting diagnoses but above all by the possibility that Davie was truly autistic, his parents were in a state of high anxiety and distress as they entered my office.

Davie was slightly rotund in the charming manner of three-year-olds. His solid physical build was normative. There was no dysmorphia (asymmetry) in his facial features that might hint at a genetic complication. Davie did not greet me with warm, direct eye contact. He kept his gaze down toward the floor, and otherwise generally avoided my eye contact. Davie's body appeared to be unusually tense, affecting his gait and, as I would later notice, the flow of his speech. Davie had a tendency to toe-walk when tense, but he "landed" when he felt more relaxed.

In the referral material his parents had noted that Davie had begun speaking late, roughly at age two-and-a-half. As an infant and young toddler, he had suffered from long-term, chronic ear infections. During my nearly twenty-five years at the Institute, I encountered similar histories among so many children. The chain reaction of developmental events related to ear infections and attendant challenges is not difficult to imagine, as noted in the case of Jack. With the auditory channel blocked because of excess fluids, a young child's hearing is compromised. The child's receptive language development would remain poor as long as fluids are a problem. The child may not respond to adults speaking to him. During that critical period of language development, the child is likely hearing the world as if he or she were under water. Not able to receive and then process verbal approaches well, it is not at all unlikely that a child would opt to play alone and apart, and might appear indifferent to auditory stimuli, which would surely sound garbled and muted. On the surface, the child might appear cut off—leading all too often to an incorrect diagnosis of PDD, AD or ASD.

As I note in other case stories, whenever I learned of chronic ear infections and ear fluids during infancy, toddlerhood and early childhood in the developmental history of a child, I usually considered the history of hearing problems "good news" of sorts, helping me in detective fashion to unravel the potential roots of the child's developmental issue. In a first visit, I considered it a high priority to invest considerable time and energy with the child's parents, to help them "replay" the development path that had likely occurred due to the ear fluids and which had led in many cases to a misdiagnosis of autism.

Chronic ear problems, hearing loss and hyperacute hearing are important clues needed in order to discern, and hopefully ultimately to reverse, the developmental chain of events that can lead to a misdiagnosis. Granted, in some cases a child might suffer from chronic ear infections and fluids and, indeed, be genuinely autistic; however, in my work at the Institute, an overwhelming majority of children whose histories included chronic ear infections, and who had experienced compromised language development, were not suffering from childhood pathology such as autism. Most had experienced an understandable delay in the development of language, with an attendant impact on personality and social functioning, yet most were not genuinely autistic in Kanner's sense of extreme emotional cutoffness. Many parents reported that when the chronic ear fluids were cleared up by the insertion of grommets or by conventional or homeopathic treatment, their child had become more responsive, and the expected stages of receptive and expressive language development then unfolded, but at a later chronological age than normal.

Davie was one such child. As his parents reported in that first session, when his hearing loss due to fluids was discovered in toddlerhood and then treated, Davie had begun to speak. Gradually, Davie began to speak with me, shyly, without making eye contact. His language was not rich, but he was able to formulate logical sentences with reasonable syntax (sentence structure) and to communicate plausibly to me—important islets of normalcy. Although shy, he was not cut off. In fact, he was sweet, warm and relational, as he began sharing his impressions about the toys with me, a stranger. He was interested, curious, verbal and communicative, and appropriately exploratory with the play materials—all significant islets of normalcy. As he talked about and related to some of the play materials scattered around the room, even en-gaging in some symbolic play, I noticed, however, the rigid, controlled, tense cadence of his speech.

When it appeared that Davie had begun to relax in what was for him a strange situation, I invited him to join me for some puzzles and games at the small table. He happily obliged—an appropriate social response. For at least half an hour, Davie engaged well with a selection of preschool learning activities, such as puzzles, picture series cards, and matching pictures with complex details. He listened with interest and responded with enjoyment as I read him the humorous storybook *Good Night, Gorilla*. As he relaxed, his eye contact at last improved.

Davie remained responsive, listening to my gentle instructions to him, and tackling each task with appropriate attention and even enjoyment. As the session continued, Davie became increasingly reciprocal, responding verbally and appropriately to our shared activities. He was not afraid to tackle these preschool challenges. It was heartening, and significant in terms of personality development, to see that he took genuine pleasure in his successes. This should not have been a surprise, as Davie's parents had reported that in his preschool, despite his mild developmental challenges, he was demonstrating excellent memory skills and proving himself to be a quick learner. At preschool he loved the presence of other children, and he was able to play simple games with them, such as chase, but he shied away from more involved cooperative play with them. Davie's delight in his successes with the puzzles and other tasks was significant. His presenting shyness seemed to be embedded in a general lack of confidence, which improved as we continued to work together.

There was an intriguing detail in his presentation. Earlier, I had noticed tension and the slightest tremor in Davie's upper body. This tremor became even more apparent when Davie sat down at the table to work with me. Curiously, this detail had not been noted in the summary reports of the several specialists who had assessed him recently in other settings. My silent observation prompted several clinical questions: A neurological problem? The residual effects of a traumatic birth? Also, to what degree was his slight upper body tremor and his tense bodily posture related to his sporadic toe-walking? Davie's speech was functional, relational, appropriate and affect-laden but at times, rather than being fluent, it sounded halting and "stuck." Were his difficulties with language fluidity also related to his bodily tension and his barely perceptible head and upper body tremor? Clearly, a neurological workup was in order, along with the attention of a skilled physiotherapist to address that bodily tension.

I was beginning to formulate an alternative understanding of Davie's presentation. Far from being cut off and autistic, Davie was underconfident and suffering from delayed development in expressive language, an observation more in line with the conclusions of two speech therapists who had seen him previously. His vocabulary and syntax were adequate but characteristic of a younger child, as might be expected from a child whose hearing had been compromised during the critical period of language acquisition. His slight social challenges in his preschool fit this underconfident, delayed language developmental profile.

He did not present with the stereotypical rocking or hand-flapping behaviors associated with autism. However, there was intermittent toe-walking, often considered an autism diagnosis clincher. While many children who are autistic (in accordance with a strict interpretation of Kanner's criteria) do in fact toe-walk, the inverse—that all children who toe-walk are autistic—is not necessarily true. This symptom alone did not have to place Davie in the shadow of an autism diagnosis. Although he toe-walked when tense, Davie was not indifferent to contact. In fact, as he edged beyond his initial shyness with me, he appeared to enjoy warm contact. His parents' report of his enjoyment of social interaction with peers in his preschool and his capacity for engaged, simple conversation in my office also negated an autistic presentation. Despite the few above-mentioned mild concerns, Davie was warm, relational, reciprocal and responsive to communication and personal connection.

Speaking in English, which Davie did not understand, I shared with his parents my impressions, based on both observation and interaction, of Davie's challenges and of his strengths. Davie, though presenting with some mild challenges, was not autistic, but rather he was suffering from delayed expressive language development, with his social challenges a by-product of the language delay, likely rooted in his earlier ear fluid problems. His overall personality, reciprocal communication and learning abilities leaned heavily to the plus side of the ledger. Although underconfident, he was not cut off. His language was not rich but he was sweetly communicative. While the negation of an autism diagnosis can be reassuring and comforting news to a parent, this simple conclusion is not enough to ensure a positive developmental trajectory. His parents would need tools, our recommendations, direction and continued support to help Davie get to a more uniformly stable developmental presentation.

At the end of this session, I shared with Davie's parents the essentials of the dynamic perspective, with its proactive emphasis on the inherent modifiability of the child. I invited them to schedule a series of further dynamic assessment appointments for Davie so that I could assess a wider and deeper range of his functioning, and assured them that the Institute staff was committed to following and supporting the progress of any child for years—in fact, for as long as the parents sought such support.

The recommendations I gave his parents were wide-ranging and reflected the multi-faceted attention that children faced with developmental challenges require. Having observed the evidence of Davie's developmental strengths, I strongly recommended that Davie remain in his typical preschool and not transfer to a special education setting as a few other professionals had recommended. His preschool teacher was warm and devoted. She also believed in Davie and in his potential, making that setting an ideal incubator for his normative development.

Davie's speech therapist also believed in his abilities, and I seconded the parents' wish to continue with her, because a therapist who believes in the latent capacities of a child is worth his or her weight in gold. I referred the parents to an excellent physiotherapist who could help relieve Davie of his intense bodily stiffness as well as provide the parents with practical exercises to do at home to help reduce the toe-walking. Finally, I explained to his parents the single most important thing that parents themselves can readily do to help a child with a receptive or expressive language challenge: Talk to your child! I urged them to speak to Davie, using a rich, developed vocabulary. They were not to "quiz" Davie by asking him questions, but to speak aloud casually about what was happening in his environment, what had happened and what was going to happen. I reminded them to speak slowly and clearly, so that Davie could absorb every word.

Sharing my initial clinical impression that Davie was not autistic and imparting recommendations were necessary at the outset, but they were not sufficient. It was clear to his parents and to me that I would need to follow Davie's progress closely over time, adding recommendations in tune with his progress, until Davie had achieved a more uniformly stable profile. We set up Davie's next appointment.

A month later, Davie returned. His parents had wasted no time in contacting the expert physiotherapist. The benefits to Davie were already evident. The degree of tension in his body had visibly diminished, his upper body tremor was less noticeable and his speech was more fluent, less withheld and less halting. The physiotherapy appeared to have relieved a considerable amount of the tension that underlay these three features. And Davie had begun playing more with friends in his preschool. His parents were still wrestling with the conundrum of whether Davie was autistic or suffering from a language delay, but they were far less overwhelmed by anxiety.

Davie himself was in a wonderful mood. No longer apprehensive in a strange situation, his greater ease was in itself an important islet of normalcy: a child who is more relaxed during a second meeting is not trapped in rigidity. He remembers and learns from experience.

Soon Davie and I were once again seated at the table, this time with more challenging cognitive activities that involved some conceptual work. With slight support he could tell me "what's wrong" in various picture cards, he could string colored beads according to a printed model, and he improved with practice in arranging picture cards to form a logical sequence story. He remained reciprocal, responsive and conversational throughout our work together, although I noticed that his vocabulary was largely concrete, lacking abstract words, concepts and nuanced emotional coloration.

The recommendations to Davie's parents at the end of this session again emphasized the importance of speaking richly, slowly and clearly to Davie, with the additional recommendation that they incorporate common concepts and words for logical groupings into their daily interactions with him, using terms for categories such as size, color, number, direction, animals, furniture and clothing. A young child's exposure to a varied conceptual receptive (comprehended) vocabulary helps ensure the child's richer expressive (spoken) language later on. Higher-level vocabulary, Professor Feuerstein counseled, was the scaffolding for higher-level thinking.

In a follow-up session one month later, Davie's use of conceptual words had clearly improved. In preschool learning activities at the table, Davie was able to tackle even more challenging tasks. He ably picked out the picture of the object that did not belong (exception) in a given group, sorted pictures into logical categories and performed well in a game that required the comprehension of the functions of various objects; for example, "show me the one we write with." Significantly, there was virtually no tension visible in his posture. I had the sense that Davie and I were building a relationship through the shared cognitive work, which he clearly enjoyed.

At the same time as his profile was strengthening toward the normative, certain behavioral problems were emerging. Davie had begun to hit his little sister. So I emphasized to his parents the importance of modeling for Davie handy little phrases which he could repeat to help him solve social/emotional conflicts verbally, such as: "Mommy, I need help" or "She's bothering me!" or "It's my turn."

Four months after his first session, Davie appeared to be undergoing a slight regression. Ear fluids had returned with a recent cold, and his body again appeared tense. In our work together at the table, I noticed that his overall tension was once again affecting the flow of his speech. Though speaking more generously, he was having word-finding problems. On the other hand, his play with small figures and vehicles, before and after our work at the table, was symbolic and expressive. Davie was open and warm in his contact with me. When I asked him an open question (as opposed to a closed "yes or no" question), "Who are your friends in preschool?" he named them happily.

In the early months of following and guiding his progress, Davie's functioning was typified by spurts of encouraging progress, along with elements of regression, such as intermittent bodily tension, or eye contact that reappeared and then waned. If a child makes dramatic progress, it is understandably easier for parents to feel secure that they are on the right path and doing the right thing. When, as is the case with most children, the child's developmental path is a mixture of progress, even breakthroughs, followed by periods of intermittently stubborn or recurrent worrying weaknesses and symptoms, the stress on the parents is very great, leading to doubts and discouragement: "Perhaps our belief in our child is not warranted. Perhaps my child is severely autistic. Perhaps we should be working according to a different model."

With a child whose path of progress climbs and descends, more frequent meetings with the child and parents are necessary, although that did not always happen. Davie's parents made a serious effort to bring him for regular follow-up meetings. My objective during each follow-up session with Davie was to qualitatively, descriptively assess the relative rate of his progress and to consider this against the vestiges of worrying behaviors that persisted or recurred. I pondered: "Was Davie drowning in a sea of symptoms?" or "Were his islets of normalcy growing and gradually coalescing into 'continents' of better functioning?" My observations, qualitative understanding of his relative progress and recommendations to his parents needed to be attuned to each developmental step forward—all are critical for strengthening, encouraging and empowering parents to continue on a process which has goal and direction; that is, realizing the child's observed, and even unseen but never-theless intuited, potential for change. Davie was making good progress, but at the same time, the need to support his parents emotionally was uppermost in my mind, since the process of any child's development inevitably involves challenges, worries, uncertainties and disappointments.

Davie's parents were able to remain stalwart and steadfast in their belief that Davie's strengths would ultimately offset his early childhood develop-mental challenges. Six months after his first appointment, his parents glow-ingly reported dramatic improvement in many areas concurrently: Davie was talking much more and his eye contact had improved significantly. He seemed more self-assured, and socially he enjoyed playing happily with friends in his preschool. The tension in his body had again receded. Behaviorally, there were fewer signs of frustration, such as hitting his sister, and he was improving in his ability to accept the limits his parents imposed.

As mentioned in other case stories, improvement in a single developmental area is always welcome and always important. However, when improvement occurs in several developmental realms concurrently—here, for example, relational, verbal, physical, social and behavioral—the significance is multi-plied. Progress in several developmental realms concurrently indicates a true shift and strengthening in a child's overall presentation.

The frequency of Davie's visits to the Institute diminished in the following year. In those few visits I observed Davie's normative cognitive growth as he moved into realms of higher-level thinking, with interest in preliminary reading and writing skills. His expressive language, vocabulary and sentence structure continued to improve. At times, vestiges of his earlier challenges, bodily tension and uneven eye contact, recurred. Adjusting our recommenda-tions to his increasing social maturity, I recommended more play dates with friends and reminded his parents to give Davie extra language processing time: "Speak slowly to him and don't pressure him to respond." With a little extra time to respond and without pressure, Davie's expressive language, as his parents later reported, fared better.

Nearly two years after his first visit, Davie's parents requested a consulta-tion to help them decide which of several regular schools would best suit Davie as he approached entry into first grade. They reported Davie's much improved expressive language and social functioning. Faint reminders of his idiosyncratic tense rhythm of speech and his slightly withheld eye contact still endured, along with episodic toe-walking, but overall his parents were con-fident that Davie could hold his own in a regular first grade class. I concurred, and recommended that of the several schools available, they select the one with the best demonstrated empathic and supportive attitude, rather than a strict and demanding setting.

Davie's parents decided not to share the history of his developmental struggles—including the reports of professionals who had once considered him autistic—with the staff of the school they selected. Davie was seen for an introductory interview at an elementary school and he was accepted on his own merit! In a follow-up phone chat with his parents several months later, his mother happily reported that his teacher was pleased with Davie's progress in school. She clearly considered Davie just another typical child in her classroom. He settled in well at that school, and for several years his parents did not return for follow-up support.

But just as Davie was about to enter fourth grade, his parents phoned. They were thinking of transferring Davie to a different school. Would I see Davie and help them with their decision? They added that Davie had succeeded socially and academically in his first three years in his regular elementary school. However, the school's academic mandate was high-achieving and too pressured, with reams of homework. Davie's parents wanted to move him to a less pressured school for typical children. And so I had the opportunity to see Davie again.

It was a delight to see how far Davie had come. A fine-looking boy now eight years old, Davie on entry to my office wanted to draw, and as he drew some surfers at the beach, he shared with me his love of water sports. He spoke about school, the subjects he liked and those he disliked. Later, he began to cry as he talked about peers who had bullied him. After the tears, Davie felt more relaxed. He smiled and laughed as he shared with me humorous exploits he had enjoyed with his friends. Davie was warm, communicative and reciprocal, with a range of typical young boy interests. I detected residues of the halting manner of speech that had characterized him as a preschooler. Initially, even in this session, his eye contact was poor. However, as the conversational exchange eased and warmed, his speech soon became more confident and fluid. His eye contact became less shy and it was nearly normative by the end of our session. Considering his sensitive nature, I agreed with his parents that transferring him to the kinder, gentler elementary school which, fortunately, some of his neighborhood friends also attended, would be beneficial to Davie. Although traces of his earlier difficulties were still evident, they were now just that—traces.

Davie was a delightful boy. He had come a long way. His parents had struggled through those early years of doubts and uncertainty about his future, when Davie's profile was more vulnerable and his progress had been uneven. Occasionally, a child's initial trajectory of progress is so dramatic that the parents can readily jettison their fears and anxieties about the autism diagnosis, and they can then focus their energies toward developing their child's perceived strengths. Davie's journey was not characterized by immediate, dramatic gain. Like that of many other children, his story is one of slow, incremental change, with periodic dips or prolonged periods of plateau followed by encouraging improvements. Davie's longer journey of several years had led to a good place—for him and for his parents.

5 Joe
Was it Too Late?

Was it too late for Joe? Fifteen years old when my colleagues and I first met him, Joe had spent his educational career since the age of seven among children and teens in educational settings designed for the behavioral training of autistic children. During his childhood, his peers at these schools, like Joe, had been diagnosed as Pervasive Developmental Disorder (PDD)—a catchall diagnosis from the era of the *DSM-IV-TR* with little clinical specificity, which was often used too generously as synonymous with full-blown autism. A decade later he and his peers would likely have been diagnosed as Autistic Spectrum Disorder.

This meant that Joe had spent close to a decade among young people whose developmental profiles were complex and impaired, and all of whom most certainly had significant difficulties in the use of language and in engaging in meaningful social interaction. Within the various schools where Joe had been placed, the predominant method of working had been behavioral modification—the use of techniques to encourage or to fade particular behaviors.

Joe's initial presentation was uniquely challenging. He appeared distracted, with a strong sense of disconnect from his surroundings. He seemed to be waiting for something to happen, for someone to tell him what to do, but Joe rarely made things happen. He rarely showed initiative, except perhaps to get a drink of water from the cooler or to go to the bathroom. He usually just sat passively, waiting for instructions.

At home with his parents and five siblings Joe was exposed to French, at school to Hebrew. So Joe lived in two linguistic worlds. His own expressive language was restricted, limited to short utterances, such as brief answers to questions that he allowed himself to hear and occasionally to respond to or requests of a concrete nature. Joe used telegraphic language to express his needs: water, food, bathroom, wanting to go home. One could not hold a conversation with Joe, as he appeared trapped within a bubble of dreamy distraction. He did not engage in conversation because he was not fully present.

Joe's language lacked emotional richness and interpersonal nuance. It would have been wonderful to hear Joe say something like "I'm upset" or "I'm bored," but these kinds of expressions were not part of his repertoire.

When my colleagues and I first started working with him, we never heard Joe say in a personal and excited way, "That was fun!" There was no personal language, no subjective vocabulary of preferences, wishes and, above all, emotion.

In speaking *to* Joe (one did not yet have a sense of really speaking *with* Joe), one sensed that Joe *might* have been listening but he was certainly not really absorbing and processing language. When he did listen, most likely his response was echolalic; that is, Joe would repeat the words he had been asked in echoing fashion. Our words did not always make it through the fog of passivity that surrounded him. Only if we spoke very loudly and persisted in speaking to him, might Joe begin to attend and respond in some way.

Joe's extreme passivity and distractedness, along with his failure to initiate, made him appear cut off. On the surface, Joe "looked like" he was autistic; his behaviors reflected the outward appearance, the form, of autism. But that was not exactly true. Joe was just somewhere else. I began to reflect on the diagnosis he had received years ago. The term PDD did not offer me any clinical clarity or insight. After the first few sessions with him, I began to understand Joe's presentation as autistiform (symptoms that "look like autism") but I did not consider Joe autistic. Something else was at work.

While his minimal expressive language was a problem, I considered his profound passivity and his near total dependence on the verbal direction of other people to determine virtually his every movement to be the crippling root of his difficulties. I interpreted his impoverished language abilities not as a symptom of autism but as a secondary effect of an undeveloped personality lacking a sense of self. Joe lacked subjective language, I believed, not because he was autistic but because he had not developed that critical sense of self.

His lack of pragmatic (purposeful), subjective, interpersonal language, his distracted cut-off stance, his tendency toward echolalia—all of these features had solidified, reinforced by years of habit. This meant that working with Joe was going to be a unique challenge. Joe was older than many other children whose stories are relayed in this book. Fortunately, Joe would be treated by the Institute's multidisciplinary staff, which included speech and occupational therapists, movement specialists, teachers skilled in Feuerstein's methods and a psychologist (my role). Although this chapter primarily summarizes what I observed during his weekly sessions in my office, the energy and strength of the team that invested in him are reflected in his story.

Joe's Early History

In early childhood, Joe's functioning had been nearly normal, with the exception of his weak expressive language abilities and the diminished social interactions associated with poor communication skills. As a preschooler, he was diagnosed with a Communication Disorder and continued for a while in regular settings. Later, at age seven, he received the PDD diagnosis and was transferred to special education settings for children considered autistic.

No doubt the staff members of the behavioral modification settings where he was placed after being diagnosed as PDD had all worked hard to cue, direct, instruct and encourage Joe to speak more and to perform better. They had succeeded, but too well. After years of being so directed, Joe had become what is called cue-dependent. He did not actively will, choose or initiate. He waited for external directions and instructions, with passivity becoming more and more ingrained in his persona. I sensed that, behind his autistiform appearance, Joe was suffering from a weakened personality that was virtually crippled by habitual passivity and the lack of a developed will.

Having spent many years in schools for autistic children that leaned heavily on a behavioral training model, Joe had learned to follow instructions: to open the door, to sit down, to sort objects into various containers, to kick a ball, to put on his coat when it was cold outside. Joe could do this. He could follow instructions. In fact he had learned to do that so well that this modality—waiting for instructions from the adult—had become an ingrained part of his personality. Joe seemed to be going through life as directed by others, but without really living it.

There is a unique word, *iatrogenic* (from the Greek word for healer), which refers to negative conditions or illnesses that result from doing what is recommended for better health: for example, a person who enters the hospital for an appendectomy, but contracts a serious infection as a result of being in the hospital. Joe's condition of extreme passivity appeared to me to be iatrogenic, a negative side effect of a skill-focused, training-based treatment direction that was originally intended to help him. Joe had learned to follow instructions and to carry out particular tasks, but the vital, emotional, communicative parts of him had atrophied over the years. So while there were parents who informed me that some programs with a behavior training emphasis had helped to jumpstart their child's progress, in Joe's case the behavioral emphasis had not worked to his advantage. A prolonged emphasis on training him, rather than on interactively challenging him, had left his developmental trajectory, in an iatrogenic manner, stultified.

Somehow, over the years, it appeared that Joe had gotten lost. Where was the real Joe, the one behind the symptoms? Behind his wall of passivity and rote communication, it looked as if Joe had simply erased himself. Where was his youthful energy, his drive to live an active, involved life? Where were his wishes, hopes, preferences? Where were his feelings, his inner world? Where were his thoughts, his abilities, even his talents? All seemed to have been swallowed up by extreme passivity and a tendency to tune out the rich nuances of the world, leaving only a tiny opening for messages that told him what to do.

I wanted to see Joe develop aspects of himself which were real, emotional, subjective, vital, alive—not mindful of an automaton. As I prepared to work with Joe, I reflected that this meant that even my vocal tone, manner of wording communication to him, and entire approach had to be completely different from what Joe was used to—that of receiving instructions, which he followed only too well by rote.

The Uphill Climb with Joe

And so, the first thing I found myself doing as a psychologist on meeting Joe was to set aside the preconceptions and misconceptions of his far too general diagnosis and to seek evidence of a completely different kind of Joe—the Joe he could have been and which perhaps he still could, at least partially, recover.

I decided to seek within him sparks of thought, feeling, and initiative in the hope that they could be ignited. I wanted to seek evidence that Joe was capable of change, and if the evidence of modifiability was not readily found, my colleagues and I would have to elicit new islets of normalcy still submerged within him. We would have to create new patterns of communication and thinking that, I assumed, had lain dormant beneath his distracted passivity. Feuerstein posited that by definition all people are inherently capable of modifiability, by virtue of their humanity. Joe was no longer a toddler or a young child. Now an older teen of fifteen, he was entrenched in self-limiting behavior patterns. Could Joe change? Could we as a team jumpstart Joe?

Joe's presentation reflected a combination of limited communication and rigidified behavior patterns, with no perseverative features other than the echolalia. This combination might have fit the now obsolete diagnosis of Asperger syndrome. However, in my estimation, that diagnosis too would have ill-served Joe because it would have potentially failed to identify that Joe's essential difficulty was existential—behind his symptoms he was lacking that vital sense of self.

I began by creating a list of Joe's presenting difficulties in an attempt to summarize them in a way that described their impact on Joe's daily functioning. This itemization was *not* undertaken in order to fit Joe into a particular diagnostic category. Rather, the list served as a mental backdrop from which I could work toward meaningful change. Joe presented with:

- A passivity that seemed to paralyze him.
- Dependence on the adult's cues.
- Inconsistent eye contact that was often avoidant.
- Lack of motivation to take initiative.
- Lack of subjective language.
- Lack of a sense of self, wishes, desires.
- Lack of a sense of humor.
- Lack of a sense of an inner world with personal thoughts and emotions.
- Frequent echolalic language, with a particular tendency to repeat verbatim any questions put to him.
- Minimal expressive language; primarily functional language.
- Language whose syntax (structure) was poor and immature.
- Lack of a sense of a unified personality.
- A strong disconnect between feeling, thought and intention.
- Underdeveloped thinking patterns.
- Limited word processing with no compound sentences.

- No cause and effect expressions (why/because; if/then).
- No evident curiosity.
- No abstract or conceptual vocabulary.
- Little associative language.
- A generally immature emotional presentation.

Within this ocean of symptoms of communicative dysfunction and lack of development of personal identity, long-entrenched over the years, it was difficult at first to discern those precious islets of normalcy. However, after reflecting on Joe's presentation in search of islets on which to build, I noted the following:

- Joe was able to speak.
- He was sometimes aware of his environment.
- He occasionally made remarks that were related to the here and now.
- He sometimes made and sustained eye contact.
- And this: Joe would generally, though not always, enter the room when I opened my office door.

This latter microscopic evidence of understanding of the visual cue of an opened door and the reading of the contextual cue—that he was meant to enter that door—accompanied by appropriate behavior, impoverished as it was for a young teen, nevertheless constituted an islet of normative functioning:

- Also, except for his verbal echolalia, Joe lacked such stereotypical behavior as flapping his hands or spinning objects. So, inversely, the fact that he lacked such stereotypical behavior became reframed in my mind as an islet of normalcy. Fortunately, Joe was not locked behind stereotypical flapping, rocking, waving or spinning behavior.

Having identified several islets of normalcy, the challenge for my colleagues and myself was to expand and strengthen these islets in his personality as well as to elicit and to create new islets of normalcy which we intuited but which were not yet evident.

Each islet of normalcy presents an opening for creative work to change and strengthen a child's profile. If Joe was passive, then our methods had to encourage activity. If Joe was cue-dependent, then we needed to devise strategies for circumventing this and for encouraging his genuine initiative. Our goal as a team was not the improvement of minute aspects or discrete skills in Joe's functioning. We wanted any particular changes to reflect a deeper, healthier, more comprehensive shift in Joe's way of being in the world. Long ago, Feuerstein had termed this kind of change Structural Cognitive Modifiability—a change in the very propensity of the individual to learn and function, a term which speaks of change in the whole person, larger and deeper than the sum of the separate elements of the individual's behavior.

We were aiming for a kind of psychological/developmental makeover—an ambitious project which some might consider unrealistic. Clearly, we understood that Joe's advanced age of fifteen meant that the process of change would be more challenging than with a very young child. Whether acquired or biologically innate, Joe's global functioning had suffered because of habit over the years. As a team, we also understood that, considering Joe's age, this "makeover" would likely not be complete. And so, when I began working with Joe, I had the sense that it did not really matter which *detail* of his presentation I addressed first. There was a need for a general existential transformation of the passive and cue-dependent way in which Joe interfaced with the world.

Beyond the sadness I felt in looking at a young teen who should have been living a full life but who had reached adolescence still emotionally and functionally a limited young child, I felt an enormous sense of challenge and the motivation to reach and to develop his personhood in place of its absence, to develop his identity and a subjective inner life where it was not yet evident, to develop subjective communication to replace his barely functional communication and to develop genuine interaction and reciprocity in place of his sparse, functional, usually echolalic verbal responses to communication directed at him.

With very young children whose ability to relate, play, speak and learn are impaired by what appears to be an autistic condition, the inspired developmental play strategies of DIR along with the vision of modifiability and the search for islets of normalcy from the Feuerstein approach usually combined to provide me with effective and creative means of bringing about change within a child's presentation. Often those early childhood DIR play strategies include sensory and kinesthetic (action, motion) games like tickling, rocking, games of chase, cause-and-effect toys and many more activities to open and close those all important circles of communication, the basic unit of reciprocity in DIR terms (Chapter 11). But Joe was fifteen years old. While others more adept at Floortime techniques might have been able to apply play strategies, I could not envision such rudimentary play with Joe.

I concluded that circles of communication from a DIR perspective, and a sense of reciprocity, from the Feuerstein perspective, had to be created without reliance on sensory infant play. Joe's sense of self and his awareness of the need for initiative and response to the world had seriously atrophied over the years, if they had ever really developed in his early childhood. His readiness to respond had been dulled by many critical years of passivity and inaction, habits that had solidified like concrete around him. I could sense that there were worlds within Joe, but it was not immediately clear how to access these as yet undeveloped worlds of thinking, relating and functioning to draw him into genuine reciprocity.

However, it was clear that in order to induce change, I would have to relate to Joe in ways which were not familiar to him, to create a kind of cognitive dissonance within him, to take him to existential places where his entrenched habitual patterns of response and behavior simply would not work, where he could not get by. That was the only way I could envision shocking Joe out of his dormancy and stretching him to respond from a genuine and more alive place, step by painful step.

Unconventional strategies began to emerge. Joe, as noted, was used to the directive way in which most adults spoke to him. The more passive he was, the more adults directed and instructed him. The more the adults determined his actions, the more passive he became. This was a useful observation and the implications of this observation extended to every aspect of my working with Joe: my vocal intonation, emotional tone, manner of speaking, manner of relating to him, session content, expectations of him—all had to be qualitatively different from a directive stance. All aspects had to communicate to him that he was a person capable of feelings and of genuine subjective responses. Our sessions had to stretch him emotionally and cognitively.

In order to counter his deeply ingrained passivity and cue-dependence, I continually attempted to create situations in which Joe would have to take initiative. I silently promised myself *never* to direct or instruct Joe what to do. The challenge was to create situations throughout our weekly sessions so that Joe would have to think in ways he had never thought before and to respond in ways which differed completely from his habitual ways of responding. My way of addressing Joe was unfamiliar to him, and at first Joe barely responded when I spoke to him. Gradually, he became attuned to a more personal and interactive mode of relating. In describing the work with Joe, I attempt to give the reader a feel for the challenges Joe presented and a sense of the strategies I used to energize him.

My tactics began at the outset of each session in the consideration of the simplest details in interacting with him. Joe usually sat outside my office waiting for me to cue him and say something like, "Open the door and come in now, Joe." More cue dependence, more induced passivity. Instead, I preferred to approach him and say something open-ended which required his inference and interpretation, such as, "We're starting now" or "It's your turn now." It was up to Joe to receive the verbal message, process it and act. If he remained seated, I moved away from him and waited at the door. It was hard not to fall into the trap of telling him what to do in order to speed up the process. I reminded myself not to open the door or direct Joe to do so. If necessary, I would just stand there and wait, until he got up and came to open the door. If he was "stuck" in front of the door, I asked him whether he wanted to continue standing or to open the door. If, for example, Joe entered the room but just stood there, I would verbally reflect that "I see you want to stand today." He was free to do so the entire session, although this did not happen. The initiative to take responsibility for his actions had to come from him.

Once inside the room, I decided from the outset to speak to him in a manner that I suspected was unfamiliar to him from his school—as a responsible, thinking individual, capable of responding and making decisions. I often began by asking Joe what he had done or had eaten the day before.

Joe usually responded in echolalic fashion, repeating my questions, "What did you do?" or "What did you eat?" I asked him questions about himself which he was completely unused to considering, in an attempt to begin building within him a rudimentary sense of genuine self. I consciously kept my tone relaxed, easy, conversational, chatty and good-humored—as far away from an instructional tone as I could muster, to force Joe to relate in a key of reciprocal communication as yet unfamiliar to him.

In this initial warm-up activity, I was looking for some genuine communication from him, and would not let up if he answered mechanically without thought or consideration. If he responded again with an echolalic "What did you eat?" I persisted in chatty fashion: "Right, that's what I asked you. I'm wondering what you had for supper last night. What kind of food do you enjoy, what kinds of foods do you really not like?" Joe did not always respond, and I did not actually force him to answer; but I did energetically repeat questions many times, expressing personal interest, and giving my reasons for wanting to know, until gradually little glimmers of response appeared. For example, Joe began to understand that I was asking him about his weekend meals. He found a solution to deal with the question. Every week he replied, "Chicken and rice." So I persevered and asked him how he likes his chicken, what kinds of salads were on the table, what he did after his meals and so on.

I continually attempted to create situations that did not lock into his expectations, in the hope that this would dislodge some block within him and that he would begin, even a little, to respond. The medium was the message: "You are not helpless. You are a person. You are here, present. I'm speaking to you as an equal. I'm waiting for an answer because I know that you, the person behind the symptoms, are capable of answering"—a fact that Joe himself did not yet know.

I avoided asking him closed questions, those which require only a "yes" or "no" answer, since closed questions made it far too easy for Joe to avoid language processing and genuine relating. Rather, I asked open questions, those which required Joe to actively process receptive language and to initiate expressive language. "How are you feeling today, Joe?" If he fired this question back in echolalic fashion, I repeated the question in a loud and cheery voice, "Yeah, I was just wondering how you're doing. I'm feeling pretty good today. How about you?"

Again, the medium was the message. The fact of an interpersonal conversation with expectations of subjective response was not yet in his repertoire. I intentionally continued in an up-beat conversational tone. Sometimes he shot back automatically, without reflecting, "Happy. I'm happy today." It sounded like he was guessing. So my next step was to challenge him. "That's great, Joe. So glad to hear that." Open question: "So why are you feeling so good today?" Eventually, over time, Joe's attention to the actual question content, his language processing and his ability to provide subjective responses improved.

The core of our sessions together often had the quality of "tough love" in order to jolt Joe out of his apathy and passivity. Sometimes in my communication with Joe, I felt like a Marine drill sergeant, not in terms of giving him orders, which I avoided, but in terms of speaking in a loud, energetic and vehement tone. As mentioned earlier, it was not clear to me how or whether I could use interactive play in Floortime fashion with this young teen. However, it was clear that the DIRFloortime goal of opening and closing circles of communication was a valuable one. Joe initially did not meaningfully open or close circles of communication—as described, he usually repeated verbal approaches to him in echolalic fashion, with no intervening language processing. In Feuerstein parlance, what was lacking was a sense of reciprocity, of two people engaged in a dialogue. It would take time.

With young childhood play activities not an evident option to me, I decided on a broad range of highly varied cognitive (thinking) activities, always with an eye toward challenging him away from rote performance, which was more comfortable for him, and toward active language processing, comprehension and expression. To present Joe with a simple puzzle or similar activity would have been to cheat him. It would have been quite easy for Joe to complete puzzles of increasing difficulty, but these would have been solo activities. Joe needed to open and close circles of communication and to engage in reciprocal communication.

Joe's receptive and expressive language abilities needed to be stretched in so many different directions that it was difficult to know where to start. I basically started from many points simultaneously, using cognitive materials that required increasingly complex and abstract language processing. For example, Joe could identify pictures of common objects ("show me the picture of the book") but this simplistic activity did not demand much linguistic or cognitive processing on his part. Instead, we worked on functional language, identifying objects by their qualities and attributes. With a range of photos arrayed on the table between us, I asked Joe questions like: "Show me the one that helps keep the room cool" or "Show me the one that's a healthful vegetable." The more conceptual or abstract the attribute, the more language processing and the more thinking Joe had to do.

Joe had not been required to develop or to use his memory, which had lain dormant and had even atrophied over the years. He did not refer to his past, or express wishes about the future. As the issue of serious memory loss in old age shows us, the loss of memory means the loss of self. So memory work was imperative not only for his memory skills per se but also for the development of his sense of self.

We often worked on personal memory in simple conversations such as "What did you do yesterday?" or "What game did you play with your little brother?" However, even focusing on rote memory, as opposed to personal or subjective memory, was important to jumpstart his memory development. We played many variations of simple memory games in which I showed Joe photos of common objects, gradually increasing the number of photos I showed him. After we had named them together, I then turned the photos over and asked him to tell me what he had just seen. At first Joe just stared.

This was an out-of-the-box thinking challenge for him. So I showed him the photos again, flipped them over, and then asked Joe what pictures we had just seen. At first he could recall the names of three objects. Four were a challenge, seven initially an insurmountable challenge. However, with time, Joe was increasingly able to look at and then recall the names of seven objects, sometimes more, whose pictures he had just seen. This was real progress. He was beginning to activate and utilize his capacity for memory and thought.

Picture sequences stories were useful to introduce Joe to the progression of time. With picture sequence stories, Joe had to arrange three to seven pictures in order to form coherent stories. This task was almost impossible for him in the beginning, but over time there was improvement. In parallel, I attempted to help him personalize and internalize concepts of before and after, past and present by asking him what he had done yesterday morning, afternoon and so on.

Tasks related to visual perception were made as challenging as possible so that Joe would have to struggle to think. I used difficult cognitive perception exercises to challenge his thinking skills. I made certain that any puzzle would be as complex and unpredictable as possible, to induce brain effort, energy and problem-solving skills.

Initially, Joe could not even relate to a question of causation ("why?"), let alone answer such an abstract question. We looked at many sets of educational/therapeutic pictures which depicted a range of social and emotional situations: for example, a picture of a young boy being ignored by his peers. I pushed Joe to give me a name for the feeling and then to suggest why the boy might feel that way. I challenged him further to tell me when *he* felt sad. Initially, identifying emotions and describing social situations were quite foreign to him. Joe lacked a conceptual vocabulary that included words for emotions, for describing objects, events and experiences and for making comparisons. He was accustomed to using the most basic, concrete, functional language. However, with persistence in our sessions, and a fair amount of energy poured into Joe, he improved. My goal was to push Joe far beyond the familiar and the comfortable. Using similar educational resources, we talked about social situations, hypothesized about solutions to social problems and discussed making decisions in the real world.

The reader may be wondering whether it was the simple repetition of activities and questions that led Joe to respond over time. I suspect not. Simple repetition of the same question of itself would not have induced change in Joe. My sense is that using materials which initially were totally foreign to Joe, continually raising the bar of expectations, energetically challenging him and insisting in tough-love fashion that Joe attend and begin to respond beyond his comfort zone, helped to move him forward.

Earlier I alluded to my feeling of, at times, acting like a Marine drill sergeant. Joe needed to be woken up, surprised and even shocked. One day, when repetition of an activity, such as recalling the names of objects in the overturned pictures, was leading nowhere, I raised my voice—not in anger, but in an attempt to awaken something in him. My tone was warm but insistent as I yelled at Joe: "Joe, you are smart. You are not stupid!" To my delight, Joe looked at me and smiled, and stood up for himself, using correct pronouns as he did so: "I'm not stupid. I'm smart!" I was delighted with his personal, subjective, well-worded response, but I continued to push him. "Right, Joe. You are not stupid. You are smart, and that's why I want you to tell me the name of two more pictures we just looked at."

After that event, when Joe was distracted, inattentive or simply unresponsive, I often raised my voice and shouted, "Joe, you are not stupid! So I want to hear your answer!" Invariably, Joe strongly agreed with me that "I am smart. I'm not stupid." In his saying these words, he was slowly building a new self-image, a conscious one. In later work with Joe, I was delighted that more than once when I presented him with a new and challenging thinking task, Joe would look straight at me *before* attempting the task and tell me, "I'm not stupid. I'm smart." This was significant communication. He had comprehended that the task before him was challenging, he had internally reflected at least a little on what this might require of him, and he was telling me that he was prepared to rise to the challenge.

As Joe's verbal responsiveness and his capacity to comprehend more abstract and conceptual language slowly improved, I continued to seek increasingly more challenging cognitive tasks. Fortunately, Joe had been taught some reading skills. I added reading comprehension exercises to his repertoire. Using some of the Institute's materials for enhancing reading comprehension, we would read a simple story one sentence at a time, while looking at the attendant illustrations. I would then ask Joe questions about the story sequence and content: "What happened after the boy fell down?" Simple questions like these stretched not only Joe's ability to think but also his ability to relate to the world.

Later in our work together, Joe surprised me one day by suggesting we do the "alphabet game," a game he must have learned, perhaps long ago, at home or at school. He demonstrated the game. He chose a letter of the alphabet and the goal was to write down as many words as possible that began with this letter. Some of his lists were shorter, some longer, but Joe could do it! While one might be tempted to dismiss this achievement as good news for a precocious first-grader but proof positive of functional retardation in a fifteen-year-old, I was delighted with the islets of normalcy his initiative represented: an improved ability to think, to use memory, to draw on his own latent repertoire of dormant early reading abilities, to suggest an activity and to share that activity. We were getting somewhere.

Yet there were some days when his combination of passivity and mental distraction lay heavy on Joe's functioning. We needed physical activity, which unfortunately would have to be limited in my small office. "Come on, Joe. Let's play baseball!" Standing apart from each other, I tossed Joe the small tennis ball which could stick to the Velcro mitts we each held. "How many times should we toss the ball to each other, Joe?" He answered and then counted as we tossed the ball back and forth. Joe's skills at catching were surprisingly good. They were also cognitively significant. In order to succeed in catching the ball, he had to focus visually and to stretch out his hand at just the right moment. Sometimes after a brief game of "baseball," Joe was energized and more likely to respond to our focused activities at my desk.

Gradually, Joe began to change. Islets of normalcy, so difficult to find at the outset of work with him, began to emerge with increasing frequency. It became clear that Joe had excellent visual perception and some good reading skills. His evidently long-ago acquired basic reading skills in Hebrew and in French began to surface more reliably. This meant that Joe possessed the ability to comprehend letters as symbols of sound that are then combined to create meaning. A colleague worked with Joe on writing notes and letters to people in his life, an activity to which Joe responded with great interest. He began sending letters to significant others and responding to the letters he received.

Joe's functional, usable intelligence improved. His thinking processes and his personal memory no longer appeared quite so rusty and atrophied. He was able to process language, including questions put to him, a little faster. His reading comprehension of short, simple texts improved. It was also evident that Joe was beginning to learn from experience, improving when various challenges were repeated. He was clever enough to announce "I'm tired!" when faced with a challenging learning task.

There were other improvements. Joe's expressive language improved from terse single-word utterances to language which was more phrasal. He even began to use sentences. After well over a year of work with him, Joe was capable of spontaneously asking a relevant question, usually concrete in nature, such as "What time is it?" We were inching toward conversation, brief samples of which occasionally occurred, with the extra processing time that Joe often required.

Joe seemed to be much more responsive in small but significant ways. His ability to use and access verbal expression appeared to be much closer to the surface. His ability to explain things, whether answers to our exercises, or to tell us what he needed to do and why, improved. Though still far behind what would be expected from a young teen, his speech nevertheless began to be sprinkled with words for feelings. He was even able to refer to his "anger" at a member of his family.

It was exciting when in the second year of our work, Joe began in modest though significant ways to initiate interpersonal communication. Joe began to show signs of appropriate emotion, such as smiling to himself when he succeeded in a task. Later, he began to display a sense of humor, with his tone expressing ironic, humorous intent of which he was clearly aware. At the outset of sessions, Joe would sometimes look at me, break into a big smile, and say with some embedded humor: "You're Shoshana!" This simple statement reflected his recognition not only of my personhood but also, and more importantly, an implicit recognition of his own personhood. Joe was beginning to develop a sense of self. In saying "You're Shoshana" he was implicitly stating "and I'm Joe!"

At the beginning of this chapter I posed the question of whether it was too late for Joe. Would Joe lead an independent life, one of meaningful work and social companionship? Even at the end of the multidisciplinary team's involvement with him, and Joe's considerable progress in many realms, that goal did not appear realistic. In another sense, however, it had definitely not been too late. He had come a very long way, shedding many layers, if not all, of passivity and disuse of cognitive and linguistic functions. His thought processes, language abilities, cognitive skills and interest in interpersonal connection had all improved, as had his sense of self.

Many years later I happened to meet one of Joe's younger brothers on the street. In response to my question of "how's Joe doing?" his brother smiled and showed me a photo on his cellphone screen. It was Joe, smiling broadly and happily, standing among a group of mildly impaired young adults and some others who were evidently their counselors. Joe was looking directly toward the photographer. He looked happy, connected and alive in his supported group setting. It had not been too late for Joe.

6 Mikey

Talk to Your Child

The most important point of guidance that I have given to parents of communication-impaired children diagnosed or otherwise considered autistic is "talk to your child." Often this is one of the first recommendations I make to parents on their initial visit to my office. And just as often, this recommendation comes as a shock to many parents: "Talk to my child? But he doesn't respond! He doesn't understand! The specialists in autism at a leading hospital told me not to waste my energy. They told me, 'Your child is autistic. He is language- and communication-impaired. He does not understand language, and he will not develop language. So don't bother talking to your child. You're talking to the wall.'" Sadly, my colleagues and I have heard many responses like these from understandably confused and distressed parents who had been so counseled elsewhere.

Already concerned about aspects of their child's development that they have noticed to be "not quite right" and hearing from a team of experts that their child is autistic, many parents can leave such an assessment meeting emotionally devastated. This is particularly true when a diagnostic report implies a pessimistic prognosis and the advice given to parents leaves little room for hope. What the child with developmental difficulties needs most is the warmth and energy of his or her caring parents. And parents need support and tools for moving forward. Shaken by the sense of finality and pessimism that often colors the diagnosis of autism, some parents, as the stories in this book attest, then suffer from a discouraged emotional state that could take them as long as several years to overcome. Precisely when the child needs mother's energetic reaching out, by playing and modeling language, mother may be less available emotionally, even withdrawing into discouragement or depression. Just when the young child needs father's warm roughhousing play and gentle words of comfort, fathers too, if influenced by inaccurate and excessive pessimism, can withdraw in their own way, distancing themselves from their fathering role, working overtime, fearing that they have nothing to give their child, or worrying that nothing can be changed even with their investment of energy. The parents of Mikey, whose story will be told in this chapter, had suffered such emotional devastation.

Inspired by Feuerstein's conviction regarding the inherent modifiability of the child, my colleagues and I loved working from a model imbued with hope of significant developmental change. Over the years, we saw so many children with autistiform and other presentations change far beyond conventional expectations. We strove to give parents the practical suggestions which we had repeatedly seen make positive differences in the face of autism-related and other challenging diagnoses. Therefore, we *always* advised, no, *urged* parents to "talk to your child."

Contrary to the pessimistic counsel of a mindset that considers autism a monolithic, incontrovertible, unchangeable affliction, the recommendation to "talk to your child" bears within it a potent message of hope to parents, but not simply hopeful as in wishfully thinking "if only." This recommendation communicates to parents that we are not about to give the diagnosis the power to determine who and what the child will become. And further, there are active steps that a parent can take to help their child who is exhibiting autistic features or who is hovering on the edge of autistiform difficulties. Often this journey toward improvement begins with a single step for the parent-child duo: "Talk to your child."

I have seen this recommendation quietly but powerfully alleviate the despair of many parents, giving them something practical and developmentally correct that they can do immediately. It has been rewarding to hear the feedback of formerly discouraged and doubting parents who report in their next visit such observations as: "I have been trying to talk to him more as you recommended. I'm not sure. But I think he is looking at me more when I talk." Or: "It's not easy talking to my child because she does not speak. I've tried to put that disturbing part out of my mind and just do what you suggested. Actually, it does seem like she's babbling more."

The most dramatic example that I can recall of the impact of this simple directive was the case of Mikey and his mother Molly. Although their sojourn at the Institute was brief, the impact of encouraging this mother to speak to her communication-impaired child was dramatic. Molly brought three-year-old Mikey to the Institute shortly after he was diagnosed as autistic at a child development center. Mikey was definitely experiencing serious communication-based developmental difficulties. He was well beyond "hovering" at the edge of developmental challenges. He did not speak, and he barely emitted sounds. He did not play. He did not make eye contact with me, and rarely and only fleetingly with his mother.

In the first of his few sessions at the Institute, Molly spoke openly, perhaps too openly in Mikey's presence, about the symptoms of clinical depression from which she had been suffering ever since Mikey had been diagnosed. Her face pale and her eyes emotionless, she seemed firmly in the grips of that depression, speaking slowly in a tone of deepest discouragement. It was not clear to me to whom I should direct my energies first—to Mikey or to his mother. While talking with Molly, I glanced at Mikey, as he wandered aimlessly about my office. It was clear that he had serious developmental problems. Yet his mother was suffering in her own way just as deeply. Crippled by depression, she barely had enough energy for herself, let alone the energy to meet the challenges of the emotional and communication needs of her communication-impaired child. Suffering from his own sense of despair and burying himself in his work, Mikey's father had delegated the care of Mikey to Molly. Molly relayed that Mikey's father had felt too discouraged and devoid of hope even to accompany Mikey to this appointment.

Given the depth of Molly's discouragement, I expended much energy as I explained to her that we viewed an autistic condition as just that—a state but not a trait, as described so succinctly by Feuerstein. A trait, I explained, is inborn, genetic and not modifiable. A state is modifiable. I drew diagrams for Molly, illustrating the difference between a more conventional way of looking at autism—as summarizing the totality of the child—as opposed to the philosophy of education and psychology of Feuerstein in which we always searched for the child behind the symptoms and the islets of normalcy that can lead to positive developmental change.

After at least forty-five minutes of attempting to plant a glimmer of hope within this despairing mother, I turned to the challenge of Mikey, who presented as avoidant on many fronts. But perhaps not all? I spoke to him gently and calmly—about what I was doing as I attempted to play with him in order to find entry points behind his serious defenses: "Oh, these are such beautiful bubbles, drifting so slowly." I silently popped a few bubbles. Was it my imagination, or was Mikey beginning to look at the lovely colors with interest? Yes, he seemed to be. I continued, sometimes in silence, sometimes making gentle "pop" sounds, sometimes talking about the bubbles and their trajectories. He definitely appeared less tense than on his entry into my office. Even this slight, almost microscopic, adjustment to a strange situation could prove to be a significant islet of normalcy.

Mikey also seemed interested in glancing at himself in the mirror. A good sign, as it was a tiny indication of interest in the world and in himself as well. Gradually, I moved closer to Mikey. He did not move away in fear. This tiny instance of non-avoidance was another islet of normalcy. I explained to Molly that I was going to try to engage Mikey in an infant game of gentle touch and tickle. Despite his slight resistance, I carefully placed him on his back on the carpet, as mother watched: baby playtime, as recommended in Floortime circles. Slowly I removed his shoes so that I could gently tickle his feet, making a special effort to seek and maintain eye contact as I rubbed his tummy or again tickled those feet.

There was a sense that Mikey was shocked at this "intrusion" into his world. But despite his occasional movements of slight resistance, Mikey, through his glances at me, was showing tiny signs of visual response. I used these islets to explain to Mikey's discouraged mother that small changes can, in time, lead to bigger ones. She did not appear convinced.

When the session concluded, I again reinforced the critical importance of her talking to Mikey. "Talk about what?" she asked. I told her to talk about what is happening around the child (activities in the environment) and within the child (feelings), and I introduced her to the Feuerstein concept of "soliloquy."[1]

Like an actor on stage, the parent, I explained, should speak to the child about what is happening—without requiring any verbal response or even eye contact from the child. Simply surround the child with the sound of the parent's voice, the rhythm and cadence of language (prosody) and, of course, words that describe aspects of the here and now.

I suggested to Molly: "For example, as you walk to the car, just talk out loud to yourself. Say things like: 'Well, we're heading to the car now. I have to find my keys. Oh, here they are in my pocket.' When you're driving, comment out loud about what you're seeing: 'What a stupid driver. He moved into my lane without signaling! We're almost home now. You're probably very hungry. I'm going to make you a yummy lunch when we go inside.'"

To head off disappointment and discouragement, I cautioned Molly that it is not easy to speak to a child who does not respond, but that this technique—of talking to even a severely communication-impaired child without demanding a response—has the potential to pave the way for later positive developmental changes. It warms up the communication channel and creates the proclivity for later language development.[2]

Molly set up a follow-up appointment for about a month later. As she left, I seriously doubted whether all the energy I had invested in trying to engage her had been effective at all. Later in the session, she looked nearly as discouraged as when she had arrived. At the end of the session, she was still voicing skepticism as to whether anything could really be done to change her child.

Three weeks later I received a phone call from Molly. As soon as she identified herself, I fully expected her to be phoning to cancel her appointment with me. But Molly had something else to communicate, "I've been talking to Mikey. Well, I guess talking at Mikey. I've been doing this a lot. And you know, it really does seem like something is different. To my surprise, he seems to be listening to me, I think. I'm not sure, but I also think his eye contact is a little better. The most exciting thing is that I am sure that Mikey has started to babble since I started talking to him a lot. I feel silly doing all this talking, but there definitely are changes in him. See you next week."

I was surprised to hear this kind of positive feedback from Molly, but I was not surprised at the changes in Mikey that Molly reported as a result of her soliloquies to him. These are the kinds of changes my colleagues and I often heard about from parents when they took the courageous and developmentally correct step of talking aloud to their child with autistic features, instead of accepting the reigning silence of impaired communication. Given the burden of her full-blown depression, I was delighted that Molly had found the strength and the determination to give it a try.

The following session, a month since his first at the Institute, I observed an important shift in Mikey's presentation. His eye contact was better—not consistent, but clearly more frequent. In that first session, he had appeared lost. Now in this second session, he appeared a bit more present—not yet attentive or relational, but definitely more present. Perhaps the most exciting change was his babbling. A month ago, Mikey's babbling had been nonexistent. Now Mikey was emitting many babbling sounds. With his onset of babbling, I could begin to coach Molly on the importance of imitation, and suggest to her ways to enhance Mikey's vocal imitation.

I warmly praised Molly for bravely launching into soliloquies and pointed out to her the importance of the small but developmentally significant changes Mikey had undergone in just a month. Were all his problems solved? Far from it. But the movement within a month from nearly non-existent eye contact to emergent eye contact, from a sense of personal absence and cutoffness to a sense of presence in the world, from silence to babbling—all these signaled that change was possible. The key variable that had changed in this past month had been his mother's speaking to him, as often and as richly as she was able to do. This had made a real difference. It was an auspicious beginning.

Understanding through this recent firsthand experience that a proactive, positive, energetic approach might offer hope of change for her child, Molly was prepared to consider my recommendation that Mikey be integrated within a nursery setting among typically developing children a year younger than him. He would likely need other therapies outside this setting, certainly some intensive Floortime from a specialist; but his inclusion within a small nursery setting of active and, above all, communicative toddlers would provide him with several hours a day of intensive "surround sound" as his younger peers would be voicing their own constant soliloquies. Together, Molly and I would have to weigh whether Mikey might need an integration assistant to help him make the most of an inclusive experience.

Molly was inclined to take this leap into educational inclusion for Mikey, but she wavered. All the other professionals with whom Molly had been in contact had strongly recommended that Mikey enter a special nursery setting among children his age, all of whom had similar communication problems and had been diagnosed as autistic. These other professionals believed that in a special setting, a "communication kindergarten," Mikey would be protected from excessive stimulation and the frustrations of a normal nursery setting, and at the same time he would receive several hours per week of various therapies that could help him. I countered to Molly that Mikey would likely develop more favorably in a regular nursery setting with an aide, immersed in the rich language, play and social skills of typically-developing peers who would serve as developmental models. Additional therapies could be provided, as needed, privately in the afternoon.

After three visits to the Institute over a period of several months, there was a perceptible thawing of Mikey's isolated, silent profile, but following those few appointments, Mikey and Molly did not return to the Institute. Several months later, Molly phoned to tell me that ultimately she had decided to place Mikey in a special education communication class. She reported that he was making progress there.

In the realities of the work with children, there was always a sense of joy among my colleagues and myself when a confluence of the child's latent potential, a parent's belief and determination, a positive educational framework, skilled and committed therapists all combined to yield exciting and positive developmental results. Thankfully, it happened often. Yet there was a sense of poignant sadness when, although we had perceived the child's positive potential to change, communicate and function, for varying reasons—some understood, some not—we did not have the opportunity to take the process of change further.

I wrestled with whether or not to include the case of Mikey in this book. The excitement of the initial subtle breakthroughs his mother had brought about simply by talking to her son was soon offset by my disappointment in not being able to follow through and support Mikey longer term to further progress. Ultimately, I decided to include his story because his mother's efforts made such a significant difference toward his developmental growth. I can only hope that Mikey grew and thrived. Despite her dark skepticism, it was Molly's courageous investment of energy to talk to her child that began to move Mikey from his detached silence. Having worked for years at the Feuerstein Institute, I knew by then the importance of not giving up on a child. But from Molly, I learned never to give up on a parent.

Notes

1 Reuven Feuerstein et al., *A Think-Aloud and Talk-Aloud Approach to Building Language: Overcoming Disability, Delay and Deficiency* (New York: Teachers College Press, 2013).
2 Ibid.

Reference

Feuerstein, Reuven, Louis H. Falik, Rafael S. Feuerstein, and Krisztina Bohacs. *A Think-Aloud and Talk-Aloud Approach to Building Language: Overcoming Disability, Delay and Deficiency*. New York: Teachers College Press, 2013.

7 Max

The Impact of Oral Dyspraxia

During one memorable winter, there seemed to be an epidemic—not of colds but of oral dyspraxia. At least six of the several dozen young children with autistiform symptoms who arrived at my office that winter for dynamic assessments were suffering from varying degrees of oral dyspraxia. All six of them had been diagnosed by various hospital child development teams, well-baby clinics or private practitioners as suffering from Pervasive Developmental Disorder (PDD) or autism. Of those six children that winter, the dramatic encounter with Max stands out with particular clarity.

Max's French-speaking parents, an impressively intelligent couple with advanced professional training, spoke openly during their first visit to the Institute of the crushing sense of despair they felt since their six-year-old son had been diagnosed elsewhere as suffering from PDD, a term which was then used virtually synonymously with autism. He had been placed in a special "communication kindergarten class" among other children so diagnosed. However, he was not thriving there at all. In fact, the staff felt he was not responding to their program of intensive therapies, and they were seriously considering recommending that he be transferred to a special class for lower functioning children.

I observed Max as he purposefully maneuvered around my office. He was a well-coordinated, proportionally built child, with no dysmorphic (asymmetrical) facial features that might hint at a genetic problem compounding his lack of language development. His eye contact was direct and expressive, with a sense of being "with it." He appeared alert and aware of details in his environment. He approached his father, seeking closeness and wanting to sit on his lap. Occasionally, he uttered vocal sounds—vowels only, no consonants. Max impressed as being very present. He did not appear cut off at all. I sensed a keen intelligence behind his overall silence. This was not the presentation of a genuinely autistic child, cut off and uninterested in interpersonal contact.

Interactive play activities using DIRFloortime strategies were not my first choice with Max because, despite his silence, he appeared so strongly present, so open to the world and so comprehending. I wanted to challenge him cognitively, but certainly the learning materials would have to be ones that did not require expressive verbal output on the part of the child, because Max was not speaking at all.

I took out my box of three-dimensional wooden puzzles, unique to the Institute, which required putting the pieces—and the frame—together such that the inner puzzle fits into the newly constructed frame. Most children loved these challenging puzzles. Max's parents looked doubtful that he could do them, but Max looked intrigued. I needed only to support him through the process of constructing the first one. After that, Max delightedly constructed puzzle after puzzle of increasing complexity. His parents were amazed, since along with the diagnosis of autism (PDD) they had been told that Max might suffer from a degree of retardation. In fact, Max was thrilled with the puzzles. He was an eager little learner, actively involved in a reciprocal process with me, signaling when he wanted each new puzzle, interpreting accurately any verbal or nonverbal clues I gave him and smiling when he finished each task. If someone had videoed this activity but had then turned off the soundtrack, an observer watching would surely conclude that Max was a completely normal six-year-old. Other than vocalizing vowel sounds, Max could not formulate words. However, he was so involved in the interactive learning process with me that it was clear that Max was nowhere near being autistic.

I decided to challenge him with more difficult cognitive activities. I reached for the booklets of testing materials for young children developed by the Institute. Known as the Learning Potential Assessment Device-Basic (LPAD-B)[1] for young learners, these cognitive challenges rely on an interactive process between learner and an involved mediator, not a detached observer. Their advantage in this initial assessment of Max was that many of the questions could be answered by his pointing to the correct picture among a choice of several. He could indicate his level of understanding with no need for speech.

I first challenged Max with an exercise that required him to select from four pictures the correct image that would complete a visual gestalt (global form). After I had showed him how to solve one or two of these, Max had no difficulty completing the others. I then presented him with a task that required making visual associations, creating a logical visual group and then finding the image that did not belong. The task required Max to select from four visual options the three best images associated with a larger picture at the top of the page, and subsequently to identify the outlier. Again Max had no difficulty with the mental operations needed for this three-tiered cognitive activity. We then moved on to sets of pictures which needed to be arranged in sequence to depict logical stories. After being helped to create one picture sequence, Max then arranged other sets of pictures to create short, logically sequenced picture stories. All of these tasks required focused attention, the ability to understand concepts such as associations, exceptions or temporal sequence, and the ability to retain mental images related to a particular concept.

Max worked extremely well, with excellent focus. He loved these challenging tasks. His parents were stunned and delighted. They were thrilled with his impressive performance, which cognitively was typical of any normally developing six-year-old. Just as his parents and I were applauding his impressive successes at the end of all these tasks, Max burst into bitter tears, weeping as if his heart would break. Throughout these tasks, Max had often tried to speak to me, looking directly at me and making many sounds. But he could only vocalize vowels, which had been impossible to interpret. He sobbed intensely for a long time, with his parents also near tears, and then finally calmed as he moved away from me and climbed into his father's lap for comfort.

His crying expressed deep sadness and terrible frustration. His parents and I could hear in his sobs how much this capable boy understood and how much he wanted to be able to speak. I stated to his parents my strong impression that Max clearly possessed a high level of intelligence. There was no hint of the functional retardation which his special kindergarten staff suspected—or of autism. My impression was that he possessed untapped intelligence above the normative, which his lack of speech had evidently obscured during processes of developmental evaluation which depended on linguistic skills, or perhaps due to failure on the part of an assessor to engage him in any way. I explained to his parents that Max appeared to be suffering from oral dyspraxia. At the end of the session, I referred them to an expert in the treatment of oral dyspraxia who had successfully treated many other children with this condition.

Oral dyspraxia describes a situation in which the child can understand language, but the hard wiring between the intention in the brain to formulate words and the muscles of the mouth, lips and tongue that actually formulate those words is flawed, compromised or essentially lacking. I sometimes explained to parents the impact of severe oral dyspraxia as follows: pretend you are asked to wiggle your ears. You understand the command and you genuinely would like to carry it out. Try as you might to get your ears to wiggle, they just won't. The muscles of your ears are just not hard-wired to your brain in a way that could make that movement possible—potentially, a very frustrating situation.

Max's parents wasted no time setting up a series of appointments with the expert. Perhaps a month after Max's visit to the Institute, I received a very moving phone call from his mother. Joyously she shared with me the news that Max had started treatment for his oral dyspraxia, and he had already spoken his first words!

My colleagues and I much preferred to conduct long term follow-ups of children with developmental challenges. However, Max's parents opted not to return to the Institute. The dramatic meeting with him occurred many years ago and, unfortunately, I was not able to contact his parents to get a much-desired update of the years ensuing. I can only hope that, once treated for oral dyspraxia, Max's first words led to his acquisition of expressive language and then the ability to read, both of which would have enabled him to begin to realize his high degree of latent intelligence. It was clear that in his special kindergarten, whose professional staff had assumed he was autistic, Max's silence due to oral dyspraxia had been misinterpreted, while his latent high intelligence had gone unnoticed. With the diagnosis redirected from autism to oral dyspraxia, my hope is that Max went on to enjoy an educational career in a normative setting.

Throughout my career at the Institute, I saw many children who suffered from lesser to greater degrees of oral dyspraxia. In some cases, the dyspraxia had already been identified, with no attendant suspicion of autism. In others, as with Max, the impact of oral dyspraxia had been overlooked, with the child's lack of speech having been misunderstood as an autistic avoidance of speech. Although my work with Max lasted for only a single session, I decided, after deliberation, to include his story because it so dramatically illustrates the tragedy of this kind of misdiagnosis. Fortunately, his story also reflects the hope that is engendered when a misdiagnosis is unmasked in an interactive evaluation, and the capacities of the child behind the symptoms are acknowledged.

Note

1 Rafael S. Feuerstein, Reuven Feuerstein, and Louis H. Falik, *Learning Potential Assessment Device-Basic: Examiner's Manual* (Jerusalem: ICELP, 2009).

Reference

Feuerstein, Rafael S., Reuven Feuerstein, and Louis H. Falik. *Learning Potential Assessment Device-Basic: Examiner's Manual.* Jerusalem: ICELP, 2009.

8 Josh

Developmental Drama

On his first visit to the Institute, Josh's serious developmental difficulties were blatantly apparent.[1] As he entered my office, I beheld a spare and vulnerable child, just over three years old, with fear reflected in his dark eyes. Josh had recently been diagnosed with Autistic Disorder (AD) at another clinic. His parents, worried and anxious, looked as if their lives were unraveling. Josh's and their difficulties had been significantly compounded by the fact that the day before his arrival at the Institute he had been expelled from his regular nursery school because of his tendency to scream and strip off his clothes whenever he felt emotionally overwhelmed.

In this new setting Josh was naturally very anxious. He clung to his mother in fear. Later, calmed somewhat, he slid off her lap. Letting Josh wander about the room so that he could find his own level of comfort without a sense of threat, I observed that his eye contact, though poor and avoidant toward me, was better toward his parents. He rarely emitted even single words, and when he did speak, it was in a barely audible whisper. His speech was marked by echolalia, the tendency to repeat echo-like what he had heard rather than to respond communicatively to the meaning of language. This echolalia was interspersed with some unclear gibberish or a kind of undecipherable speech (random vocalizations or sound making). There were no stereotypical perseverative movements, despite his latent tension. Early in the session Josh did not attempt any purposeful or symbolic play with the toys laid out on the carpet.

After only a short time in this new setting with a stranger, anxiety flooded him. He began to cry and scream. In one deft move he peeled off his shirt and opened my office door. He continued to scream as he ran through the corridors, undressing as he fled. His mother dashed after him, scooped him up and brought him back, panicked and overwhelmed.

Given his level of fear and anxiety, and since both his parents were in the room to restore his sense of security, I felt it best to lock the office door to provide passive containment of his overwhelming anxiety. His parents readily gave their consent to locking the door. This was done to limit him safely and to allow the door to "do the talking," so that I would not have to actively restrict him by telling him "no" repeatedly. Naturally, locking the door initially induced his further anxious screaming, but ultimately it served to contain his fear. Drawing comfort from his parents' hugs and soothing tones of voice, Josh began to calm. By the last thirty minutes of this two-hour initial assessment session, Josh had calmed enough to begin to explore some of the toys on the floor—a tiny but significant step away from his panicked sense of fear and toward meaningful mastery and expression by means of play.

Josh sat down on the carpet beside a tiny dollhouse equipped with furniture and human figures. He looked through the windows and doors of the doll-house for several minutes. As he explored, Josh quietly mumbled to himself, with occasional audible gibberish or a barely decipherable word. Sensing an opportunity for nonverbal contact with him, I quietly lay on the carpet in such a way that it was possible to make a little eye contact with Josh from the opposite side of the dollhouse through its windows. He peered at me cau-tiously through the little windows. His eye contact was fear-laden but direct. So as not to overwhelm this highly reactive and fearful child, I decided to keep words to a minimum; my vocal tone remained soft, measured and gentle in order to keep his anxiety level down. Silently initiating a play idea, I arranged little chairs around the tiny table on the "lawn" in front of the dollhouse. Josh began to play! He quietly sat some tiny figures on the chairs and in the faintest whisper said, "birthday party." Josh possessed symbolic understanding! The child figures seated together had triggered a fleeting but emotionally mean-ingful association and had prompted verbal expression.

This session, so fraught with Josh's terror, was a challenging start. I was observing Josh through several lenses: Feuerstein islets of normalcy, DIR circles of communication and play therapy. Years of training and clinical experience in play therapy had helped me to remain calm and centered through the storm of his fears. After the storm, Josh was slightly more ac-cessible. Experience with play as the language of the child gave me confidence that if there was any way to reach beyond Josh's panic, it would likely be through play and not through verbal interaction, at least initially. The play-based developmental model of DIR provided me with a kind of internal mantra as, throughout Josh's distress, I kept thinking, "Look for opportunities to open and close circles of communication. Try to make contact with Josh." My many years at the Institute had grounded me in the understanding that a child's initial presentation, what he or she appears to be, is not a reflection of what the child can yet become. And so, I was looking for evidence of changeability of his initial symptoms. Even microscopic evidence of change can be meaningful: islets of normalcy in a sea of symptoms.

Josh's islets of normalcy were subtle and small, but they were there. Josh had shown that he was capable of calming when supported and soothed by his parents—awareness of relationship. He even sought comfort by approaching them. By the end of the session, he had achieved enough calm to be able to use play materials in a meaningfully expressive fashion. And his play con-tained welcome symbolic understanding! After the storm, I noticed that actual words were embedded within his gibberish. And despite his high level of anxiety and tension, which can often translate into perseverative stereotypical hand-flapping and other such behaviors, Josh did not present with any stereotypical repetitive behaviors. Rather, his presentation appeared to be rooted in his highly sensitive emotional reactivity, possibly compounded by sensory issues, evident in his peeling off his clothes when distressed.

Had I been evaluating Josh by using conventional means of autism symptom check-lists or the *DSM-IV* or *DSM-5* criteria, Josh's poor eye contact, echolalic language and general paucity of purposeful play behavior might have nudged him toward a PDD, an AD or an ASD diagnosis. But by using the perspectives of emotionally receptive and developmentally grounded interactive play, within a context of belief in the inherent modifiability of the child, the prognosis for this child behind the symptoms was far more encouraging.

Josh's and his parents' most pressing problem, however, lay beyond the confines of my office. Josh had just been expelled from nursery school because of his tendency to scream and undress when emotionally overwhelmed. I advised his parents to avoid placing him in a special nursery for communication-impaired or autistic youngsters, as had been recommended at another clinic. The tiny islets of normalcy I had observed indicated a more promising developmental direction. I suggested instead that they look for a small home-based nursery setting with a warm caregiver and just a few children. Yet there was one niggling question: with his high degree of reactivity, and his tendency to scream and undress when stressed, how long could Josh last in a new setting without some extra help?

Although for most of the children in this casebook, play-based DIR strategies coupled with the search for islets of normalcy sufficed to launch meaningful dynamic assessment and treatment work, Josh's extreme degree of emotional reactivity together with his severe lack of confidence indicated that Josh would require some preliminary work from a different direction, if there was to be any hope of his adjusting to a new nursery setting.

With his parents' enthusiastic agreement, I offered to launch a trial series of six play therapy sessions with Josh. I suggested to his parents that we re-evaluate Josh's progress after this trial run. In keeping with basic play therapy practice, the goal of these sessions would be to provide Josh with a safe and protected space in which to express through play the intermingled rage, fear, panic and sadness which so often flooded him. Hopefully, a short-term intervention would serve to troubleshoot the intensity of his panic reactions and stabilize him enough to be able to adapt to the new nursery setting. Fortunately, this hypothesis proved correct. The next six sessions, with child-centered play as their focus, helped move Josh along.

In the first of these weekly sessions, Josh clung to his mother, who sat opposite me at my desk. With his mother's consent I again locked the office door to keep Josh and his fears contained. Clasping his mother, Josh cried and screamed for twenty-five minutes, during which time I sat calmly and tried to appear nonthreatening. When Josh's sobs subsided, I quietly placed a couple of teddy bears on the desk. Josh looked at me and angrily flung one of the bears to the floor. It was an opening! Thinking "nonverbal empathy" from my play therapy background and "circles of communication" from the DIR model, I flung the other teddy bear in mock anger to the floor after him. Josh smiled—a promising opening of a circle of communication, a lovely islet of normalcy and a flash of contact between us. I brought out more stuffed animals. Josh began flinging these, too, as I offered them to him one at a time. Sometimes I also took turns "angrily" throwing the stuffed animals. Josh smiled more frequently and began to calm markedly, clearly enjoying this reciprocal play activity and "empathy through action" rather than through words. There was a sense of movement in this session.

A week later, Josh again began his session by crying while clinging to his mother. However, this time he cried for only ten minutes. When he calmed, I brought out the stuffed animals. Josh knew what he wanted to do. Soon we were taking turns flinging animals all over my office. Josh really warmed to this activity. So out came dozens of miniature plastic animals; and these, too, we flung all over the place. Josh calmed further, evidently encouraged by the fact that his latent rage was not overwhelming the therapist. Nonverbal participation in his play evidently had communicated enough of a sense of emotional safety to enable Josh to become a little more relational.

It seemed safe to add verbal elaboration to our activities. I decided to speak for him, reflecting his feelings in the first person rather than the second person; in a sense, taking on and expressing for him his rage and fear. As I flung some of the animals, I said softly in mock anger, "Yuck! I don't want this crummy bear." Josh brightened. It seemed safe to go a little further. "I'm mad and I don't want this dumb tiger!" Josh continued to calm. My verbally assuming and voicing his intermingled difficult feelings served to legitimate and mitigate those feelings.

Flinging little animals around my office became our play focus for four more sessions. During the last of these sessions, Josh felt secure enough to climb off his mother's lap and to again explore the dollhouse and its furnishings. This time, he did so with more confidence, talking and even singing to himself, with improved eye contact toward me, and more frequent, audible speech.

Meanwhile, Josh's parents and the caregiver in his new small nursery setting had reported dramatic improvement in Josh's overall presentation and behavior shortly after the first three toy-flinging sessions. Josh was calmer, warmer and more relaxed at home, with far fewer temper tantrums. Though still anxious, as when parting from his parents in the morning, Josh was coping better and beginning to notice the other children in his nursery. He had started playing in parallel fashion alongside his peers. On one occasion, he had become flooded with fear and had peeled off his clothes in his new nursery, but the caregiver handled this event gently and supportively. Josh was able to calm and to return to the nursery activities. His undressing behavior never recurred.

In parallel with these mood improvements, Josh began to speak more and in a more audible tone. His vocabulary improved and his sentence length grew incrementally. His mumbled gibberish diminished. Josh's parents excitedly reported that he was beginning to show interest in symbolic play with small figures at home.

Following this series of play sessions, Josh and his parents participated in follow-up visits, at first once every few weeks, then monthly, and then with decreasing frequency as Josh improved and his progress stabilized. For about a year during follow-up sessions, the focus remained on building Josh's symbolic play skills and on strengthening his ability to express himself using words.

As Josh improved in these areas, the focus of the work shifted toward the primary mandate of the Institute, that is, to the cognitive realm. A much-improved though still powerful little personality, Josh at ages four and five was very intelligent—enough to seek to avoid any learning tasks that emphasized his weaker verbal skills rather than his highly developed perceptual skills. Gradually, Josh's cooperation and functioning on more challenging cognitive tasks improved. His parents then sought the help of an occupational therapist expert in sensory integration exercises, whose intervention unlocked tension and advanced Josh markedly. After one month of daily massages and eye-hand coordination work by the parents as coached by the occupational therapist, Josh's speech and language blossomed further.

My recommendations to his parents throughout a follow-up period of several years were far-ranging and reflected the broad range of disciplines that must be taken into consideration when helping a developmentally challenged child improve. I provided guidance on how to mediate effectively according to Feuerstein theory, specifically the need to speak with Josh richly, slowly and clearly, emphasizing key words in tune with the Feuerstein method of soliloquy; on DIR techniques for supporting his rudimentary symbolic play; on the importance of limiting video, computer and television hours; on the necessity of ensuring that he had many symbolic play materials on which to scaffold language development; on the potential usefulness of supplementing conventional medical treatment with qualified alternative intervention for his frequent ear infections; on Josh's need for "play dates" for social skills practice; and on the importance of maintaining Josh in a typical school setting, supplemented by therapies as needed in the afternoon.

Often an early diagnosis of AD, PDD or ASD, like a menacing shadow, trails even the child who has emerged from his difficulties. This was certainly the case with Josh, who at ages five and six was speaking in clear sentences, participating in kindergarten activities, reading fluently and learning ably, although still experiencing mild difficulties with peer contact. Josh's parents had told his kindergarten teacher about Josh's earlier diagnosis. It was necessary for me to speak with this teacher several times in order to reassure her that Josh should no longer be considered autistic and that he was fully capable of further normative growth. It was difficult for this teacher to let go of the no longer applicable diagnosis and to enjoy Josh in his own right. Ultimately, his parents transferred Josh to a more warmly receptive educational setting.

By the age of nine, Josh was a highly competent fourth-grader, active in after-school activities and well-liked by his friends. Josh and his parents then disappeared from the Institute radar. Many years later I happened to meet Josh's parents on the street. They happily updated me. Now twenty years old, Josh had enjoyed a successful academic and social career in high school and was currently busy continuing his education and a normal young adult social life. The fearful child who had first entered my office at age three, meeting many of the formal criteria for an autism diagnosis—avoidant eye contact, severe expressive language difficulties, lack of social adaptation, and panic-tinged sensory/emotional reactivity—had achieved a totally normative profile.

A trial series of play therapy sessions had initially precipitated an intensification of Josh's emotional symptoms in my office, but this safe and protected space soon helped him establish a basis of trust and confidence in the therapist and, above all, in himself. The safe and protected space of the therapeutic playroom, combined with Floortime strategies for circles of communication and imbued with the Feuerstein belief in the imperative of the modifiability of the human being, along with the supportive presence of his mother, had all helped Josh begin to build confidence and ego strength. Once Josh was stronger emotionally, he was able to progress to more developmentally complex goals associated with learning, and to enjoy a healthy normal social, academic and professional life. The shadow of a restrictive diagnosis no longer menaced him.

Note

1　A different version of Josh's story appeared in a chapter by the author entitled "Barriers, Bridges, Breakthroughs: Play Work with Autistic Spectrum Children" on pages 77 through 110 in *The International Handbook of Play Therapy: Advances in Assessment, Theory, Research, and Practice*, edited by Charles Schaefer, Judy McCormick, and Akiko Ohnogi, published in 2005 by Jason Aronson of New York. Parts of that chapter have been revised and are reprinted herein with permission.

Reference

Levin, Shoshana. "Barriers, Bridges, Breakthroughs: Play Work with Autistic Spectrum Children." In *The International Handbook of Play Therapy: Advances in Assessment, Theory, Research, and Practice*, edited by Charles Schaefer, Judy McCormick, and Akiko Ohnogi, 77–110. New York: Jason Aronson, 2005.

Part II

Theoretical Groundings

The developmental paths of Jack, Sasha, Annie, Davie, Joe, Mikey, Max and Josh—all with their varying presentations—share commonalities. All of these children were originally diagnosed as autistic (AD, PDD or ASD). For each of these children, an autism-related diagnosis had misrepresented their particular developmental challenges and/or masked their unique potential. Part Two on Theoretical Groundings will present the concepts, descriptive terminology and related reflections and considerations that helped to create a qualitatively attuned clinical milieu which enabled the latent strengths of children with autistiform symptoms to become manifest.

The first theoretical model, by educational psychologist Reuven Feuerstein, emerged from the world of cognitive development and offers the clinician a uniquely grounded perspective regarding human potential. Chapter 9 summarizes Feuerstein's impressive life's work and then presents his key concepts that helped to catalyze our work with children who presented with autistic features, terms such as modifiability, reciprocity and islets of normalcy. The notion of islets of normalcy proved so essential in qualitatively assessing and treating children with autistiform symptoms that two chapters are devoted to the concept. Chapter 10 defines and describes islets of normalcy, illustrating their usefulness in the assessment process of two very different children. DIRFloortime, which evolved from the realm of infant mental health, is the second model presented (Chapter 11), with a summary of the essentials of Greenspan and Wieder's DIR developmental stages and a sampling of the recommended play activities helpful in transporting the child in autistiform isolation toward relationship and communication. Chapter 12 revisits the concept of islets of normalcy, and describes how the sensory-based questions that underlie Floortime practice can serve as guidelines for identifying many islets of normalcy. Three case examples in this chapter help bring this synthesis to life.

Chapter 13 uses a conceptual magnifying glass and examines, in the spirit of a close reading, the diagnostic criteria for autism within the *DSM-IV-TR* and *DSM-5*. The discussion grapples with some of the challenges embedded in those criteria. Chapter 14 highlights the case for a more generous use of the term autistiform in the assessment and treatment of children who present with symptoms that appear, on the surface, to represent an autistic condition. Chapter 15 argues for the need for a paradigm shift, away from the confines of an autism diagnosis–focused paradigm and toward descriptive, qualitative work in order to actualize the child's potential beneath the autistiform symptoms. Chapter 16 presents concluding reflections.

A parent or practitioner accustomed to relying on conventional means of symptom-focused assessment might at first experience a sense of unease when shifting toward working in a qualitative paradigm of play interaction, emphasizing the child's strengths rather than symptoms, and setting the autism diagnosis aside while adopting as a goal an active encounter with the child and his or her latent potential. Hopefully, the chapters following will make movement toward such a paradigm shift more feasible.

9   Feuerstein's Vision and Vocabulary

Professor Reuven Feuerstein was a man of vision—inward vision, into the latent potential of each individual—and more. Highly knowledgeable and well informed in the fields relevant to his life's work—cognitive development, child development, genetics, neurology and psychiatry, to name just a few—he was intuitive, original and brilliant in formulating unique terms, methods and materials that again and again proved effective in advancing the cognitive (thinking), learning and general developmental functioning of a vast range of special populations.

It is difficult to capture in words the sense of energetic hubbub that characterized the work atmosphere at the Feuerstein Institute in Jerusalem. When I first arrived in 1992, it was housed on two modest floors of a small apartment building. Children with special needs and their parents, from Israel and all over the world, waited in the halls, literally for hours, for an appointment with the Professor, anxious to get a second opinion about their child's difficulties, potential and prognosis. Professor Feuerstein used his observations and interactions with these children as teachable moments, calling particular staff members to come to his office "Immediately!" to observe, to learn from his perceptive comments, and to offer their own perceptions and ideas for assisting the child. Back in the narrow hall, staff members and the children they had just assessed using Feuerstein's unique dynamic assessment materials spilled out of the inadequately small offices. In fact, there were not even enough offices for the number of people on staff. It was a variant of musical chairs! After getting over the shock of such a situation, it was not long before I, too, learned to knock on an office door and plead with a colleague, "I have to assess this child. Please could you write your report on the enclosed porch?" It was madness, but there was something in it of the primordial chaos of creation. The lives of people with special needs, young and old, were being changed for the better, often dramatically.

Two years after I arrived at the Institute which the Professor had founded two generations earlier, we moved to larger quarters. The chaos diminished, but the atmosphere of creativity remained. It seemed that the number of programs and the number of staff people just expanded to fill the larger space. The same sense of brimming energy, along with a great sense of purpose—mission even—transferred to these new quarters.

Just walking down the halls of the Institute, now expanded to five floors, one encountered Down syndrome children, who were integrated in regular schools, heading for the Professor's office to show him the new words they had learned to read, or brain-injured accident victims wheeling themselves to instructional sessions because the Professor's unique methods and materials had proven effective in restoring damaged brain functioning. There were children and youths between the ages of six and nineteen with genetic syndromes, retarded functioning, developmental delays, severe autism and even psychiatric problems heading out from the Institute's school for severely impaired young people for an outing in the nearby park. There were young adults with special needs milling about the lobby. Some were participating in the Institute's program to prepare them to work in restaurant kitchens or as aides in geriatric care facilities. Higher functioning young adults with Down and other syndromes were enrolled in the Institute's course to prepare them for marriage. Professor Feuerstein's commitment to extracting the maximum potential from each individual was total, and it extended across the lifetime.

In the halls, one might also encounter management executives from the fields of business and industry who had come to relay to the Professor how his materials for cognitive development were being used to strengthen workers' problem-solving abilities, with clear benefits to overall performance. There were cadres of psychologists and educators from Israel and around the world who came to learn Feuerstein's theories and methods so that they could apply them in the educational systems of their home settings. There were representatives of local universities who had agreed to accept the results of Feuerstein's dynamic assessment methods in admitting applicants from impoverished, educationally deprived backgrounds to medical school. Though these applicants' scores on conventional medical school entrance tests had been insufficient for acceptance, Professor Feuerstein, his son Rafael, and other key staff members convinced these university representatives that the results of dynamic assessments had shown that it was the challenges of cultural deprivation, not a lack of intellectual abilities, which had accounted for their lower scores on conventional measures. These young medical school applicants, they argued, had demonstrated in the process of dynamic assessment that they had the cognitive abilities needed to succeed in medical school. And they did!

One was equally likely to encounter any of a number of renowned world experts from the fields of education, psychology, psychiatry, medicine and so on with whom Feuerstein shared warm professional relationships. And, pertinent to this autism casebook, it was in this way that I was introduced to Serena Wieder and the DIRFloortime model which she and Stanley Greenspan had developed.

Later in this chapter, I will introduce Feuerstein's unique professional vocabulary and highlight the way these terms were helpful in assessing and treating children thought to be autistic. But first, it is worthwhile to learn about the roots of this charismatic man whose tireless, inspired and inspiring work continued until literally the day he died at the age of nearly ninety-three.

Roots

Professor Reuven Feuerstein began his pioneering work in the field of psychology in Europe immediately after World War II, assisting orphaned children who had been traumatized by their wartime and concentration camp experiences. Even before completing his formal studies, Feuerstein perceived flaws in the conventional, normed intelligence and aptitude test results that were being used to determine these children's future placements. Those results had indicated that these scarred postwar children were functionally retarded. The Professor recognized that trauma and the resulting developmental interruption in their lives, not an inherent lack of ability, had impacted on these children's test scores, skewing the results toward retardation and obscuring their latent capabilities, which he discerned. Dissatisfied with assessment instruments which stressed *performance*—that is, the need for the learner to produce specific bits of knowledge rather than encouraging the development of thinking *processes* in a focused, relational, interactive context— Feuerstein began creating interactive, dynamic assessment methods without norms, and later cognitive development materials which stressed the processes of learning and thinking in the relational context he prized. The refinement and wide application of these methods and materials became his life's work.

Feuerstein undertook his postwar master's studies as a protégé of Piaget, later completing a doctorate in psychology at the Sorbonne. He then struck out in his own unique direction, stressing the intrinsic modifiability of the human being. As the reader has already encountered in the teeming halls of the Institute, his lifelong work touched a remarkable range of special needs populations of virtually all ages and types who came to the Institute from all over the world: Down and other genetic syndromes, those considered learning disabled or functionally retarded, even gifted underachievers.[1] Over the course of his lifetime, that range of populations extended to include his groundbreaking work with brain-injured and stroke victims. Later, he encouraged the development of revolutionary materials to enhance the cognitive faculties of the blind.[2] Current research on brain plasticity, which verifies changes in brain cells and brain neurotransmitters as a result of the intensity and type of external stimuli, scientifically substantiates what this forward-looking psychologist proposed two generations ago—that brain cells are modifiable and respond to the stimuli of the environment. For Feuerstein, it was an "I told you so" experience. To have had the opportunity to participate in the process of extending the impact of his vision, theories and methods to children thought to be autistic was a gift—to the children, to their parents and to my own growth as a psychologist.

The Vocabulary of a New Language

When I began working at the Institute carrying out postdoctoral research in autism, I had to learn two new languages: Hebrew, and the unique professional vocabulary of the Feuerstein Institute. The latter was more challenging for me! Veteran staff members were talking about modifiability, potential, mediation and deficient cognitive functions. There was more: input, elaboration and output phases of cognition; dynamic assessments, Instrumental Enrichment. It was foreign and overwhelming at first. I learned to speak Hebrew before I learned to speak Feuerstein.

I had just finished a four-year doctoral program in Canada in counseling psychology, specializing in play therapy. I loved working with young children, helping them heal emotionally and behaviorally when feelings of sadness, fear or anger overwhelmed them. It was not an easy transition from the world of feelings to the Feuerstein world which focused on cognitive development. But I already spoke the language of play and knew how deeply play could reach into the essence of a child. Ultimately, play provided the bridge, a way of linking the Feuerstein paradigm to my deepening interest in autism.

I was not always able to connect the dots, that is, to apply all of the Feuerstein vocabulary to my work with children who presented with autistic-like symptoms. However, his concepts were there, in the air, the energy and the mission of the Institute. They were an essential part of the fertile ground from which grew the Institute's unique qualitative way of assessing and treating these children. And for this reason, I wish to share the basic elements of this new professional language that I learned. Wherever relevant, I link these terms to their applications to my work with children originally thought to be autistic.

Modifiability

All the branches of Feuerstein's remarkable body of work are deeply rooted in a single concept: human beings, by definition, by virtue of their essential humanity, are modifiable.[3,4] Simple? Simplistic? Superficial? Wishful thinking? None of the above. Rather: Complex. Challenging. Consequential, and requiring a combination of determination and vision to discern latent abilities, and much hard work to bring those abilities to actualization.

Feuerstein called this inherent capacity for modification Structural Cognitive Modifiability (SCM), a somewhat cumbersome term. It means that the very propensity—a combination of willingness, openness and ability—of the human being for thinking (cognition), and other developmental capacities, can be modified. Long before the current interest in what is known as brain plasticity, he concluded that significant modification of cognitive abilities was possible because the human brain was capable of change and adaptation.[5,6] He understood that human beings can change even beyond initial expectations when the environment *anticipates and promotes* such change. You have to want and believe in that change, and then work hard toward it.

> You must have a need that something should occur. When you have that need, you will believe that change is possible. With that belief you will search for ways to create change, and not rest until you have found them.

You will discover that with sufficient commitment and energy, the ways exist. You will act to make it happen, convince others to follow you, and ultimately change expectations and systems of wider scope.[7]

Feuerstein's focus on modifiability refers to more than acquiring a specific skill, such as learning to count or to read or to speak in sentences. It means that a fundamental change in the orientation and openness of the learner toward learning or thinking in general can be brought about by effective mediation with the learner. He anticipated that the results of his unique assessment methods would create not scores and norms but what he called a "profile of modifiability,"[8] a functional, descriptive profile of the child's (or adult's) challenges and strengths.

There is something philosophical, spiritual perhaps, about psychological or educational work that is rooted in a belief that human beings are intrinsically modifiable. When working in the trenches from this perspective, the thinking goes something like this: "This child has Down syndrome, but I can see unexpressed and unexplored abilities to be developed." Or: "This child cannot read, but calling the child dyslexic seems limiting to me. I'm going to try many creative methods to get to the roots of this child's difficulty and to bring this child to reading ability." Or: "This child appears autistic, but I see evidence of strengths and get a sense that the symptoms are weaker than they appear at first glance. This child is capable of making substantial progress."

So the first step is vision, seeing the potential behind the diagnosis, then anticipating a process of modifiability behind the presenting symptoms and impairments, then working hard to attain it. Even with children or adults who came to the Institute for dynamic assessment or therapeutic intervention, and whose latent potential was difficult to see at first, Feuerstein and his staff nevertheless intuited—believed—that more robust potential was present. It had to be, because before us was a human being, intrinsically capable of modifiability.

Did this mean that someone who initially presented as functionally retarded might eventually attend university? No, although there were cases where this in fact occurred, to the absolute shock of other professionals. Did this mean that a child with Down syndrome would shed all signs of this syndrome? No, but thousands of children with this syndrome were helped to achieve educational/developmental goals originally considered beyond their reach, and were able to go on to enjoy fuller, richer lives than more conventional schools of treatment had ever considered possible. And then, there were children like Sasha, Annie, Davie and Josh, who initially presented with autistiform symptoms, who shed or markedly diminished any autistic-like symptoms, and who continued on a normative or near-normative developmental path. We believed that the potential was there. We sought it. And when we could not see it, we worked hard to elicit it and even to create new facts on the ground. A belief in the inherent capacity for modifiability of the child with autistic features definitely propelled the work.

Feuerstein's commitment to catalyzing *modifiability* in the cognitive abilities of even the most challenging presentations was directly transferable to our work with children with autistic features. But with these children, the focus was primarily on the modifiability of their communication and relationship capabilities. I looked for evidence of modifiability in the way the young child with autistiform symptoms meets, greets, relates to and communicates with the world. Without these prerequisites of *being* in the world, learning skills would have had little meaning. Mikey (Chapter 6), for example, in his first appointment appeared detached and cut off until our bubble and tickle encounter. By his second appointment, after his mother had begun to speak with him, his eye contact had improved and he had begun to babble. More importantly, he just seemed more present and less detached. Something basic within him had begun to shift.

Mediation, the Mediator and a Modifying Environment

Feuerstein believed that the abilities of a person were not solely, or even primarily, determined by the dictates of genetic makeup, physiological impairments, age or even the assumptions deriving from a given clinical or diagnostic category. He agreed that these external factors certainly *can influence* development and functioning, but he believed, and substantiated this belief with his life's work, that the intentional and warmly interactive (reciprocal) focused input, *mediation*, by a mediator has the power to mitigate and even override many genetic, diagnostic, prognostic and similar "givens" to create meaningful change within the individual.[9] Mediation is not the same as "top-down" teaching. The mediator is not looking for the child to produce bits of information or even to supply correct answers. Instead, the mediator is trying to encourage more active, focused and efficient cognition. Intentional, reciprocal human interaction, in his view, was the key.

Professor Feuerstein prioritized the impact of what he called a modifying environment—an environment that anticipates, supports and works for changes—over hereditary factors, stating famously: "I will never give the chromosome the last word."[10] While never denying the influence of biological factors, true to this latter assertion, he and his staff worked to provide the modifying forces, the mediation, that would help extract the maximum potential from even the most challenging developmental situations.

Feuerstein's optimistic belief system is not a naïve one. Changes in a child do not appear magically. He understood that people develop in part according to the expectations imposed upon them but mostly because of the energy invested toward those expectations. The results are so dependent on the quality of the energetic mediation of the mediator. This meant much hard work. Feuerstein expected as much from his staff as he did from himself. If a child was not speaking, speech development still remained a goal: "Use creative ways to bring the child to speech!" If a child had poor eye contact: "Use all creative modalities to engage eye contact!" If a child did not yet point, a basic building block of attending to the world: "Create the ability to point!" If the child did not imitate sounds, words or behavior: "Teach this child to imitate!" Feuerstein knew that the child's ability to imitate is the foundational skill for future learning.

The notion of *mediation*, the convivial, energetic interaction between adult and child/learner, was readily transferable to children with autistiform symptoms. Instead of mediation which relied on cognitive materials, the mediation for these children relied on the power of developmental play. Although Feuerstein's foundational theories did not include attention to play, the Institute, which valued the energetic pursuit of the individual's latent abilities, proved to be a warmly compatible setting in which I could adapt the developmental wisdom and the play-based strategies of DIRFloortime when working with children diagnosed as autistic.

Young children whose social communication problems were more prominent first of all needed to build important prerequisites for being in the world, as congruent with the DIR developmental ladder (Chapter 11): calming and attending (emotional regulation), pleasure in emotional connection, eye contact, expressive language, symbolic play. So the mediation to encourage reciprocity and connection with these young children took place by using play materials and activities. These efforts at mediation initially strove to enhance the child's sense of being in the world, and later attended to their cognitive abilities.

Input, Elaboration, Output

Feuerstein had a gift, among many others, for conceptualizing what he was doing and why he was doing it. He divided the learning experience into three phases: input (taking in information), elaboration (processing information) and output (communicating what one knows/understands). For each phase he identified many deficient cognitive functions. These were never thought of as learning disabilities. They were simply the specific points that helped the mediator focus efforts to help the learner, for example, the need for attention to detail, the need for facility with concepts, or the need to decrease verbal impulsivity.

Because my play-based interactions with young children with autistic features were focused more on the child's emotional, relational presence than on what and how they were learning, the notion of deficient cognitive functions figured less in my work. But the general notion of the input, elaboration and output phases was very relevant and helpful.

For example, children with autistiform features are often diagnosed, at least partly, by their problems with verbal output, such as lack of or minimal speech. As I explained to many parents, often the child's problems lie more in the realm of input. That is, information is not coming out (the child is not talking) because it is not getting in (the child is not attending/receiving). And that is one of the reasons that our advice, "talk to your child," was so important. Rather than trying to squeeze words out of the child (output), we were trying to jumpstart the basic attention to spoken language (input) in many children like Jack, Sasha, Annie, Davie, Joe, Mikey and Josh.

Materials for Modifiability and Dynamic Assessment

If Feuerstein's ideas had remained only in the realm of theory, they might have been wrongly dismissed as simply wishful thinking. But his powerful and unique concepts led to his developing qualitative, descriptive, process-oriented instruments for assessing learning potential, and materials for developing what he called metacognitive abilities, such as conceptual fluency, abstract thinking, problem-solving and many other cognitive skills. Throughout his lifetime he continued to develop many ground-breaking cognitive development materials.

His Learning Potential Assessment Device (LPAD),[11] for example, consists of varied and challenging cognitive tasks which provide opportunities for the assessor to interact with the learner's thinking processes, and to qualitatively, descriptively note the difficulties and the improvements which occur during the testing itself. The LPAD, and its offspring the LPAD-Basic (LPAD-B)[12] for younger children, attend to perceptual, conceptual, logical, problem-solving and other cognitive skills. Some items are scored, but if scored they are neither normed nor related to an IQ score.

In the supportive, interactive style of dynamic assessment, when using these materials, the focus is on the *process* of thinking and learning with understanding, not the *product* in the form of a correct answer. The goal of dynamic assessment, as noted, is to pursue and demonstrate change within the individual during the assessment itself. The atmosphere during assessments is relaxed and supportive.

There were many other brilliant materials, but developmentally the young children with autistiform symptoms were not yet ready to tackle them. Feuerstein's Instrumental Enrichment (FIE) tools[13] comprise a veritable library of booklets, each geared to develop, in the presence of a skilled, trained mediator, a foundational cognitive skill, such as making comparisons, understanding opposites, spatial orientation, temporal relations and many more concepts. Other cognitive enrichment materials were also developed to address particular cognitive goals, such as reading comprehension,[14] memory improvement[15] and inferential thinking[16] or to assist the cognitive developmental needs of unique populations, such as the blind.[17] Over several generations, many pertinent research studies have confirmed the efficacy of the methods and the materials that Professor Feuerstein and his Institute produced, materials which are now used in over seventy countries.[18,19,20]

The concept of dynamic assessment was wonderfully applicable to young children who presented with autistiform symptoms. With these young children, the use of sensory-based and other play activities, rather than dynamic assessment materials, yielded rich and relevant information about the difficulties, and more importantly, about the strengths (islets of normalcy) and degree of modifiability of many children behind those symptoms. The vision of inner potential, the interactive style of working and the goal of qualitative understanding were the same as with the LPAD assessment materials. Only the medium, play materials and activities, differed.

Many of these children first needed playfully elicited prerequisites of relating and communicating before their cognitive potential could be targeted. Enter play, which provided the medium and the milieu for assessing and treating them. Play-based interactions with these young children yielded rich descriptive details of even the minutest transformations in communicative and/or relational interest and abilities. In fact, the play activities with young children served as a dynamic assessment and treatment intervention concurrently, because during a play-based dynamic assessment, my colleagues and I were already working to effect change.

Consider, for example, Sasha (Chapter 2) and Mikey (Chapter 6), who were similar in their degree of presenting isolation. Each had a huge developmental backlog of sensory, relational and communication difficulties that needed to be addressed before enhancing their cognitive functioning. Gently rocking Sasha in front of the mirror or blowing bubbles with Mikey were not simply sweet activities to do with developmentally challenged toddlers. These activities were the very stuff of assessment and treatment together!

The complex, challenging instruments of the FIE booklets were usually far beyond the intellectual reach of the younger children with whom I worked. The LPAD, too, was pitched considerably higher than the abilities of the toddlers or young children I assessed, although sometimes the Basic versions of the LPAD or FIE could be used with the higher functioning young children who already possessed some key developmental prerequisites. That is, the child was verbal, relational and developmentally ready for preschool cognitive challenges.

An aside here about the use of such materials with older children who present with autistiform symptoms is appropriate. With children roughly eight years old and over who presented with wooden, rigid or restricted communication styles, as typical of Asperger disorder in the past, it was enjoyable to use the LPAD materials in ways that challenged the children's communication patterns. I would add a healthy dollop of energy, warmth and especially humor during assessments to help stretch these children beyond their communication comfort zone toward warmer, more personal and more relaxed communication. For example, during the "getting to know you" part of the interview before diving into assessment materials, I might challenge them: "You mean you like onion pizza better than plain pizza? Are you kidding me?" Or during assessments: "You're amazing! How did you know that this answer solves the problem better than that one?" The LPAD materials were the medium. The essence of the assessment for older children with rigid communication patterns was the quality of our communicative exchange.

A Roadmap for Progress: Four Phases

Without norms, how does one chart a child's progress? By paying attention to detail and by using rich qualitative description. Feuerstein provided a conceptual roadmap for charting the child's progress. He described four phases of transformation that lead from the absence of a positive, efficient cognitive or developmental function to its tentative appearance, and then to its growing relative strength in a child's profile. In the first phase, a cognitive ability such as attention, perception or logical thinking might be completely absent, nonexistent in the child's profile. In the next phase, the child has improved so that the particular cognitive ability is embryonic and visible, but just barely, in the child's profile. In the third phase, the presence of the ability is more frequently seen, but it is fragile, in an unstable state, easily extinguished. In the final phase, the skill, ability or quality is prevalent in the child's profile and it is firmly entrenched. These phases do not provide the clinician with a diagnosis, an IQ score or a norm. But they do provide an enormously useful roadmap for the qualitative process of growth and the realization of potential.

An example from the cognitive realm: a child might at first completely lack the capacity for visual attention to a printed page; after much mediation, that child might show embryonic, emergent visual attention skills. After more hard work, visual attention might occur more often but it is still fragile, easily extinguished within the child's profile. Finally, that skill or capacity has an established presence in the child's skill repertoire. The child is now reading or doing worksheets.

When engaging a child with autistiform symptoms, these four phases related to the emergence of abilities—*absent, embryonic, fragile (episodic) and established*—were extremely useful as conceptual guidelines. Although I did not point them out in the case stories in this book, they were always present as mental scaffolding, quietly guiding my work. They helped me qualitatively gauge the transformation of a child's symptoms from seriously autistiform toward a more normative presentation. For example, Sasha's lack of eye contact at age eighteen months transformed to episodic eye contact, to increased eye contact though still fragile in his overall profile, to entrenched, stably relational and reliable eye contact by age three. With regard to speech development, within the month between his first two sessions, Mikey began to move from a lack of consciously expressive sounds to occasional intentional sounds, to emergent babbling. It would have been a delight to accompany him to the next phase of imitative approximations of words. Josh, well beyond babbling when he arrived, quickly moved from gibberish with embedded episodic words to purposeful speech. The goal of the work was to help the child with autistiform features trace a path which followed Feuerstein's phases from the absence to the stable presence of various developmental capacities.

Following that Road

Feuerstein's unique theoretical vocabulary, as well as his hands-on involvement in offering his counsel whenever we requested it, continually inspired, illumined and guided our work with children with autistiform symptoms. When qualitatively evaluating the purported accuracy of an autism diagnosis with which the child had arrived at the Institute, honing in on communication and relationship variables initially outweighed seeking evidence of efficient cognitive functioning. Using warmly supportive interaction (mediation) in a process of qualitative, descriptive dynamic assessments with the autistic population, while incorporating play materials and play activities as the very substance of the assessment, proved to be an ideal way to encounter the difficulties of a communication-impaired child and to uncover the child's strengths. As these case stories relate, so often when we did so we found that symptoms that at first appeared intransigent began to show signs of flexibility. This helped in understanding whether the autistiform symptoms on the surface were typical of genuine autism (when using a strict interpretation of Kanner's primary criteria) or not.

As the Institute's work with children with autistic features developed over the years, Professor Feuerstein increasingly came to adopt the term *islets of normalcy* in our qualitative assessments of the children and our treatment interventions with them. The concept of islets of normalcy proved enormously useful in applying Feuerstein's vision to children with autistiform symptoms, as the following chapter elaborates.

Notes

1 Reuven Feuerstein, Yaakov Rand, and Rafael S. Feuerstein, *You Love Me!! Don't Accept Me as I Am: Helping the Low-Functioning Person Excel* (Jerusalem: ICELP, 2006).
2 Roman Gouzman, "Tactile Instrumental Enrichment: IE Program for Blind Learners," *Educator* 12 (2000): 30–37.
3 Reuven Feuerstein, Pnina S. Klein, and Abraham J. Tannenbaum, *Mediated Learning Experience (MLE): Theoretical, Psychosocial and Learning Implications* (London: Freund, 1991).
4 Reuven Feuerstein, *Theory of Mediated Learning Experience: About the Human as a Modifiable Being* (Tel Aviv: Ministry of Defense, 1998).
5 Reuven Feuerstein, Rafael S. Feuerstein, and Louis H. Falik. *Beyond Smarter: Mediated Learning and the Brain's Capacity for Change* (New York: Teachers College Press, 2010).
6 Reuven Feuerstein, Louis H. Falik, and Rafael S. Feuerstein, *Changing Minds and Brains: The Legacy of Reuven Feuerstein* (New York: Teachers College Press, 2015).
7 Louis H. Falik, *Changing Destinies: The Life and Times of Prof. Reuven Feuerstein* (Bloomington, IN: Xlibris, 2019), 160.
8 Mandia Mentis, Marilyn J. Dunn-Bernstein, and Martene Mentis, *Mediated Learning: Teaching, Tasks, and Tools to Unlock Cognitive Potential* (Thousand Oaks, CA: Corwin, 2008).
9 Reuven Feuerstein, "Shaping Modifying Environments through Inclusion," *Transylvanian Journal of Psychology*, Special Issue no. 2 (2007): 9–23.
10 Reuven Feuerstein and Antoine Spire, *La Pedagogie a Visage Humain* (Paris: La Bord de L'Eau, 2006).
11 Reuven Feuerstein, Yaakov Rand, and Mildred B. Hoffman, *Dynamic Assessment of Retarded Performers: The Learning Potential Assessment Device, Theory, Instruments and Technique* (Baltimore, MD: University Park Press, 1979).
12 Rafael S. Feuerstein, Reuven Feuerstein, and Louis H. Falik, *The Learning Potential Assessment Device-Basic: Examiner's Manual*, Second Revised Edition (Jerusalem: ICELP, 2009).

13 Reuven Feuerstein, Yaakov Rand, Mildred B. Hoffman, and Ronald Miller, *Instrumental Enrichment* (Baltimore, MD: University Park Press, 1980).
14 Rafael S. Feuerstein, Reuven Feuerstein, and Louis H. Falik, "Learn to Ask Questions for Reading Comprehension," in *Feuerstein Instrumental Enrichment Basic Program: User's Guide* (Jerusalem: Feuerstein Publishing House, 2009), 132–42.
15 The materials for enhancing memory functioning are currently being refined by Rafael S. Feuerstein and are not yet published.
16 Rafael S. Feuerstein, Reuven Feuerstein, and Louis H. Falik, "Know and Identify," in *Feuerstein Instrumental Enrichment Basic Program: User's Guide* (Jerusalem: Feuerstein Publishing House, 2009), 112–18.
17 Gouzman, "Tactile Instrumental Enrichment," 30–37.
18 Alex Kozulin et al., "Cognitive Modifiability of Children with Developmental Difficulties: A Multi-Centre Study Using Feuerstein's Instrumental Enrichment-Basic Program," *Research in Developmental Disabilities* 31 (2010): 551–59. This reference and those in the two notes following are intended to be representative of the large number of studies that have researched the efficacy of Feuerstein's methods and materials.
19 Daniel D. Kurylo et al., "Remediation of Perceptual Organization in Schizophrenia," *Cognitive Neuropsychiatry* 23, no. 5 (2018): 267–83.
20 Cecilia Smeraldi, Giulia Mazza, and Liana Ricci, "Feuerstein's Instrumental Enrichment in the Treatment of Obsessive Compulsive Disorder: A Preliminary Study," *Cognitivismo Clinico* 12, no. 2 (2015): 111–22.

References

Falik, Louis H. *Changing Destinies: The Life and Times of Prof. Reuven Feuerstein.* Bloomington, IN: Xlibris, 2019.

Feuerstein, Rafael S., Reuven Feuerstein, and Louis H. Falik. *The Learning Potential Assessment Device-Basic: Examiner's Manual*, Second Revised Edition. Jerusalem: ICELP, 2009.

Feuerstein, Rafael S., Reuven Feuerstein, and Louis H. Falik. "Know and Identify." In *Feuerstein Instrumental Enrichment Basic Program: User's Guide.* Jerusalem: Feuerstein Publishing House, 2009.

Feuerstein, Rafael S., Reuven Feuerstein, and Louis H. Falik. "Learn to Ask Questions for Reading Comprehension." In *Feuerstein Instrumental Enrichment Basic Program: User's Guide.* Jerusalem: Feuerstein Publishing House, 2009.

Feuerstein, Reuven. *Theory of Mediated Learning Experience: About the Human as a Modifiable Being.* Tel Aviv: Ministry of Defense, 1998.

Feuerstein, Reuven. "Shaping Modifying Environments through Inclusion." *Transylvanian Journal of Psychology*, Special Issue no. 2 (2007): 9–23.

Feuerstein, Reuven, Louis H. Falik, and Rafael S. Feuerstein. *Changing Minds and Brains: The Legacy of Reuven Feuerstein.* New York: Teachers College Press, 2015.

Feuerstein, Reuven, Rafael S. Feuerstein, and Louis H. Falik. *Beyond Smarter: Mediated Learning and the Brain's Capacity for Change.* New York: Teachers College Press, 2010.

Feuerstein, Reuven, Pnina S. Klein, and Abraham J. Tannenbaum. *Mediated Learning Experience (MLE): Theoretical, Psychosocial and Learning Implications.* London: Freund, 1991.

Feuerstein, Reuven, Yaakov Rand, and Rafael S. Feuerstein. *You Love Me!! Don't Accept Me as I Am: Helping the Low-Functioning Person Excel.* Jerusalem: ICELP, 2006.

Feuerstein, Reuven, Yaakov Rand, and Mildred B. Hoffman. *Dynamic Assessment of Retarded Performers: The Learning Potential Assessment Device, Theory, Instruments and Technique.* Baltimore, MD: University Park Press, 1979.

Feuerstein, Reuven, Yaakov Rand, Mildred B. Hoffman, and Ronald Miller. *Instrumental Enrichment*. Baltimore, MD: University Park Press, 1980.

Feuerstein, Reuven and Antoine Spire. *La Pedagogie a Visage Humain*. Paris: La Bord de L'Eau, 2006.

Gouzman, Roman. "Tactile Instrumental Enrichment: IE Program for Blind Learners." *Educator* 12 (2000): 30–37.

Kozulin, Alex, Jo LeBeer, Antonia Madella-Noja, Francisco Gonzalez, Naama Rosenthal, Ingrid Jeffrey, and Meni Koslowsky. "Cognitive Modifiability of Children with Developmental Disabilities: A Multicenter Study Using Feuerstein's Instrumental Enrichment-Basic Program." *Research in Developmental Disabilities* 31, no. 2 (2010): 551–59.

Kurylo, Daniel D., Richard Waxman, Steven M. Silverstein, Batya Weinstein, Jacob Kader, and Ioannis Michalopoulous. "Remediation of Perceptual Organization in Schizophrenia." *Cognitive Neuropsychiatry* 23, no. 5 (2018): 267–83.

Mentis, Mandia, Marilyn J. Dunn-Bernstein, and Martene Mentis. *Mediated Learning: Teaching, Tasks, and Tools to Unlock Cognitive Potential*. Thousand Oaks, CA: Corwin, 2008.

Smeraldi, Cecilia, Giulia Mazza, and Liana Ricci. "Feuerstein's Instrumental Enrichment in the Treatment of Obsessive Compulsive Disorder: A Preliminary Study." *Cognitivismo Clinico* 12, no. 2 (2015): 111–22.

10 Searching for Islets
of Normalcy

An atmosphere of pessimism and fatalism seems to hover over the field of autism. As the stories in this casebook relate, all too often, upon seeing a young child in my office for the first time, a child who had been elsewhere diagnosed as autistic, PDD or ASD, I encountered the fear, anxiety, and even despair and grief of the impact of this diagnosis on many of the parents. If the parents had received written reports from one or more professionals, or had gleaned information about autism on the internet, they had often already encountered highly discouraging prognoses regarding their child's challenging presentation. The diagnostic process which most parents had experienced with their developmentally delayed or challenged child characteristically focused on identifying and quantifying (occasionally qualifying) symptoms which had led to their child's being considered autistic and therefore, it was assumed, impaired—often with a prognosis that was reminiscent of someone who has learned that they have a terminal disease.

In tackling the challenge of assessment and diagnosis of children who appear to be autistic, rather than focusing on the evident symptoms, Professor Feuerstein adopted the term "islets of normalcy." Within the ocean of the child's difficulties and symptoms—the compounded impairments in language, communication, relational and social abilities—these islets are the examples within the child's behavioral, emotional, functional repertoire of non-symptomatic behavior, in a sense the anti-symptom.

These islets of normative behavior might be microscopic, fleeting and infrequent within the child's overall profile and behavioral repertoire. But they are always *significant*. For example: a child whose eye contact is almost non-existent who suddenly looks directly at mother when she begins to sing to him; a highly avoidant child who suddenly takes father's hand to open the door; or a child without language who suddenly hums a recognizable melody. In a more conventional mode of working, one of seeking symptoms, these miniscule nuggets of developmental promise are often overlooked. In the Feuerstein worldview, they are prized.

When working within the perspective of Feuerstein, we are always on the lookout for islets of normalcy when we observe any child. This is particularly true with children thought to be autistic. When we observe such a tiny islet, we ask ourselves, "How can I expand and strengthen this islet?" not in the behavioral modification sense of primarily increasing its frequency, but with the aim of weaving and then firmly establishing this expanded and strengthened islet into the totality of the child's personality. If an islet, perhaps of rudimentary communication, does not yet exist, then the goal is to *create* islets even when they are not yet evident, by using creativity, play, music, movement and play-based cognitive tasks to elicit new islets while continuing to expand and strengthen existing ones.

The concept of islets of normalcy is important throughout the course of assisting a child initially considered autistic, but it is perhaps most critical in first meetings with such a child and his or her parents. This is so because characteristically, as noted, most parents arrive weighed down by the diagnosis which may or may not be accurate and burdened by their own assumptions regarding prognosis gleaned from their own reading or from various professionals. In a first session in particular, a positive focus on identifying and even creating islets of normalcy has the power to create a paradigm shift that can positively affect parental attitude, morale and actions, and which may dramatically impact on the treatment plan and prognosis of the child.

The impact on the child, as the clinician actively, playfully and meaningfully interacts with the child in order to explore, elicit and magnify the microscopic evidence of more normative functioning, is no less dramatic. In my office, children not infrequently began to make eye contact, communicate in some fashion and function more meaningfully. While the islets I observed may have been evanescent and fleeting, they were nonetheless present—and they subsequently informed further work with the child, the practical recommendations to the parents and even the child's future educational placement.

This chapter presents descriptions of the first sessions of two young children, each of whom had previously been diagnosed elsewhere as suffering from autism. In each case, the clinician's focus on islets of normalcy, rather than the very evident symptoms, led to just such a paradigm shift, for the caregivers and for these two children. Over the years, there were many other children for whom our focus on islets of normalcy moved the prognosis away from pathology and toward normative functioning, often dramatically so. In the cases of Ernie and Sammy presented here, I have attempted to give the reader the feel of the actual process of the clinician's searching for islets of normalcy.[1]

Ernie

It was two o'clock in the afternoon, and I was facing my last session of the day at the Institute, after a wearying morning working with a number of challenging children. So I was not feeling enthusiastic as I pulled out the file of the new little boy, now six years old, who had been diagnosed as autistic at the age of two by a well-known Israeli specialist in autism. I looked over the specialist's report included in the referral material. Over the course of several sessions, the specialist had applied the criteria of the *DSM-IV*, then in use, in addition to observing the child at play and conducting an interview with his foster parents. The specialist's conclusion was unequivocal: Ernie was autistic. The attendant report was only too rich with supporting descriptions of the child's lack of speech, his lack of communication and lack of ability to develop relationships, and his impoverished cognitive functioning, which the specialist had concluded was typical of a child suffering from retardation. The specialist had recommended that Ernie continue in a special educational setting intended for autistic children, a small class in which he would receive several hours of therapy per week, but be placed among similarly impaired children who lacked language, social, communication and play skills. Feeling even wearier after reading this pessimistic report, I braced myself for a challenging and difficult last session, one which would surely require massive energy output to assess such an impaired child. I opened the door of my office to Ernie and his foster parents. I was not at all prepared for what ensued.

A bright-eyed and eager little boy, with sparkling blue eyes and fetching blond hair, burst into the room with a warm and enthusiastic smile. For a second or two, he looked at me directly with eyes that spoke of anticipation and which communicated a sweet and energetic little soul. Could this be the same child described in the specialist's report? Ernie was very present, not at all distant or cut off. There was something absolutely charming about him. My mood lifted. The afternoon was going to be quite different from what I had imagined a few minutes ago, when I had been strongly influenced by the mood, tone and conclusions of the specialist's report.

Ernie was one of my earlier clients at the Institute. I have since learned, when reading reports from other specialists, to reserve judgment and to be highly cautious of conclusions and recommendations when previous testing of autism was based on tallied formalized criteria and/or when it was clear from the report that the specialist, or team of specialists, had not played with the child or otherwise actively and warmly tried to elicit engagement. Even in the face of a stack of reports which expressed a negative prognosis of a given child's abilities, I sought to explore each child's potential and come to my own conclusions about the child's abilities.

"Let the child explore. Don't interfere with a child's initiative and explorations especially in an initial session." This was a cardinal rule for Reuven Feuerstein whenever he first observed young children in his office, and he had taught us well. Feuerstein's emphasis on permitting a developmentally impaired child, or so suspected, a free range of behaviors and expression (without compromising safety of course) within an assessment or treatment situation resonated strongly with my background and training in play therapy.

A child's initiatives and explorations in a new setting tell us an enormous amount about how a child sees and relates to objects, activities and people in the setting. The observation allows us, of course, to note where a child's development is challenged or compromised, but more importantly, it allows us to gather an impression of the parameters of the child's weaknesses and to identify initial evidence of the child's strengths. It is not enough to note symptoms. We must identify the energies, strengths and capacities that each child possesses in order to overcome or, at the very least, to modify and mitigate these weaknesses.

A child's weaknesses, developmental deficits and various difficulties, incidentally, should not be used against him to confirm a pessimistic fate, but should rather be considered a kind of "baseline," not in the sense of behavioral intervention, but in the sense of galvanizing our own energies to help this child move toward meaningful change: "This is the child's starting point. Now, let's see how we can modify and improve this profile." So the early part of an initial assessment session with a young child suspected of experiencing a developmental difficulty such as autism was always devoted to letting the child move about freely, handle objects, make noise, play at will or even just sit mutely on the floor.

Letting the child lead, without structuring the contact by requiring the child to sit at the table and "perform" too early on, helps to reduce the child's anxiety. In an atmosphere of implicit support and acceptance of a child's initiatives, the child can feel a bit more in control in a strange setting and in the presence of a total stranger. The less anxious a child feels, the more likely it is that we, as clinicians, will see the child at his or her best and most capable, rather than impeded, impaired or even frozen with fear and anxiety. All too often throughout my career, I heard from parents about the distressing experiences they and their children had experienced in previous assessment procedures elsewhere which had involved, at least partially, observation of the child and parents by a team of professionals—social worker, occupational therapist, speech therapist, psychologist and perhaps psychiatrist—sometimes with an entire assessment team observing the child within the same room. What child would not freeze with dread in such an inhibiting situation?

A close reading of the child's uninterrupted interface with a new setting and its contents and people can yield much rich and important developmental information. I signaled to Ernie's foster parents to remain quiet and assured them that it was fine if Ernie handled the play materials or moved about the room in any way he wished.

As Ernie wandered around my office examining the few play materials I had scattered around the room, he was explorative but he did not meaningfully engage or play with any toys. Both aspects were significant. On one hand, he was curious and had an appropriate sense of exploration in a strange setting. On the other hand, there was no meaningful play development with a given object. Some might be tempted to conclude that his lack of purposeful or symbolic play was an autistic-like feature. While a restricted repertoire of play behaviors could indicate an autistic-like feature, there are other possibilities. The child's inner world may be underdeveloped. The child may be lacking experiences of warm, caring play interactions with his caregivers. The child may feel inhibited in a strange setting. It is so important to view a particular behavioral facet in context and to spread as widely as possible the net of possible explanations for a behavior. It is critical to use extreme caution and *not* to assume that a particular behavior which "fits" the official autistic criteria necessarily means that the child is autistic. There are multiple potential meanings to every behavior—and not all of them point to developmental pathology.

Soon Ernie stopped wandering and stood opposite me as I sat at my desk, where I was paying close attention to possible indicators of developmental challenges. But I was seeking far more than that—because the identification of "symptoms" is not the end game in the work of child development, education and psychology. Identifying symptoms is only the beginning. Far more critical in assessing young children is identifying those sparks of relevant functioning, such as incipient and even latent communicative intent, and the child's hesitant, sometimes even microscopic, attempts at reciprocity and relationship. When we are seeking evidence of the capacity for healthier functioning in a child, we must actively search for even the smallest "islets of normalcy" in the vast sea of the child's symptoms.

Symptoms, quite frankly, can often be rather obvious. Even a casual observer can readily see that a child "is not speaking" or "has poor eye contact" or "does not communicate or engage in relationship." To engage solely in a mission of seeking symptoms is to shortchange the child's present latent abilities and his or her future capacity to change. Beyond and behind the symptoms, we clinicians are duty bound to seek evidence of the child's latent ability to communicate, play and learn. Once we identify these islets of normalcy, we can work to enlarge, expand and strengthen them within the child's profile. Slowly we work to assist these tiny specks of normal functioning to grow and coalesce. As the islets coalesce into a larger body, the proportional impact of the symptoms diminishes as the child's strengths grow. This is a fact which I have witnessed many hundreds of times with children as the result of the hard work of parents, my colleagues and myself began to bear fruit.

In quietly observing Ernie, I had already noticed a number of islets of normalcy:

•   His energetic and eager burst into the room. Evidence of enthusiasm.
•   His brief though clearly direct look into my eyes, which communicated energy and emotional presence.
•   His curiosity and purposefulness.

On the deficit side of the ledger, he was not yet playing with the objects with pleasure. I made a note of this as something important to work on—pleasure in play and meaningful play expression.

When Ernie wandered over to my desk and stood opposite me, I quickly pulled out a colorful picture book. He looked at me. More islets!

- He had moved over to my desk of his own volition. Indication of interest in relationship. Communicative intent. Curiosity perhaps.
- Further evidence of capacity for direct eye contact.

I noted that Ernie was drooling ever so slightly. Oral hypotonia likely, I thought. This weakened oral musculature might be affecting his severely delayed and impaired speech development. To this point, Ernie had not yet spoken in my office. There was the possibility that his lack of speech was attributable not to autism but to weak oral muscle tone. In his case, oral hypotonia might be good news, with what had been considered autism a secondary result of a primary deficit—often correctible with the appropriate type of speech therapy.

Ernie took an interest in the book I showed him. He spoke! "Tree." "Dog." "Man." Nearly seven years old, Ernie was making initial utterances typical of a one-year-old child. Some clinicians might be—and in his case had been—quick to critique such impoverished speech as evidence of possible autism and even mental retardation. But I was looking for islets of normalcy and Ernie's few words were potent with relevance:

- Ernie had shown interest in the pictures in the book.
- He had identified the objects by name.
- If he could utter words, then he possessed the capacity for speech.
- He uttered these words in relationship to my intervention. Ernie was now engaged in a reciprocal learning activity of looking at pictures in a book.

I was intrigued and excited to get these glimpses of the charming child behind the very symptoms which had been so well documented in the referral report. Ernie did not understand English. So I engaged his long-term foster parents in discussion in English about his background, which they had already described in their referral material. Ernie was the middle child of three. Because his parents suffered from complex emotional difficulties, they could not meet his needs. This had led to his transfer to foster care. While not an islet of normalcy, this contextual information supported the understanding that Ernie's early years had been characterized by a lack of nurturance, serious developmental under-stimulation, a compromised capacity for a warm and meaningful parental relationship and even suspected aggressive discipline toward him.

Ernie's devoted foster parents relayed more. They expressed their anguish that Ernie had been placed by the educational system in a very low func-tioning special kindergarten for autistic children: "We believe that he is in-telligent. He has been living with us for a long time and we see evidence of his intelligence in all kinds of things. And he's started to speak recently." These caring people had intuitively noted on their own accord many islets of nor-malcy which they relayed to me.

I had already seen enough islets of normalcy and sparks of purposeful communicative intent to sense that Ernie possessed much more potential than the report by the specialist had described. Ernie had begun to participate with me in the semi-structured, reciprocal activity of looking together at a picture book, so I felt it safe to change the atmosphere and to move from the un-fettered observational stage of this first meeting to attempting a more struc-tured, cognitive and goal-directed activity.

I invited Ernie to join me at the little table as I pulled out some puzzles suitable for a preschooler. Ernie readily focused on these and enjoyed doing them.

- Ernie understood and responded to the invitation to sit by the table. Evidence of relevant language comprehension and awareness of a social cue.
- Ernie was interested in structured tasks.
- He was capable of task orientation, remaining interested and on task.
- His ability to concentrate and his attention span, as I sat beside him expressing interest and encouragement, were quite good.
- The simple puzzles were proving too easy for him. Evidence of a lively intelligence.

Seeing that these puzzles were not a challenge for him, I pulled out my box of three-dimensional wooden puzzles, unique to the Institute. They consist of an inner puzzle of perhaps three to five interlocking pieces, symmetrical or asymmetrical, set within the frame of a small wooden box, which itself has to be constructed by the learner. These puzzles require motor planning skills and the ability to work on two planes—the inner puzzle needs to be turned and inserted into the three-dimensional box frame constructed around it.

I scattered the pieces of one of the simpler ones on the little table and showed Ernie a completed box puzzle. Ernie was stymied. He had no idea how to construct all these scattered pieces into a whole. A more conven-tional view of cognitive capacity might have surmised at this stage that he was "impaired" or "retarded." But in the dynamic interactive method of assessing and helping learners of all ages, as developed by Feuerstein, the critical question is not "Can the child do it or not?" but "What interactive mediation will enable the child to move from 'not knowing' to 'knowing'?" In other words, if I give this child the mental or verbal tools and the strategies to learn, can he internalize these? The question then becomes, not "does he know?" but "can he learn?" I wondered, and set out to explore this question with Ernie.

I decided to demonstrate for him the construction of a simpler three-dimensional puzzle. I verbalized my actions as I sat by his side and con-structed the puzzle that had overwhelmed him, explaining to him, "This circle goes inside the square. Now the square fits inside the diamond. Now I slide them along the table and grasp them all together with my hands, like holding a sandwich. Now they need to fit inside this piece, which looks like a bed. Now the piece that looks like a window slips over them, and finally this goes on top."

Ernie was enthralled. He then readily did the puzzle on his own.

- Ernie had watched and listened to my demonstration with rapt attention.
- He readily benefitted from the demonstration and the voiceover description.

But had he learned or was he simply imitating without understanding? I brought out another three-dimensional wooden puzzle. Ernie constructed it with ease.

- Ernie was capable of genuine learning, that is, of generalizing what he had learned when presented with another example.

Yet something else was happening. Ernie was thrilled and excited with the challenge and the fact that he had done the puzzle readily. He cried out eagerly, "More!! More!!"

- Ernie was hungry to learn.
- He possessed intrinsic motivation within a learning process.

That afternoon, I brought out my entire selection of at least fifteen such puzzles for Ernie. He did them all—enthusiastically, even joyfully. Occasionally he had difficulty with the more complex puzzles, but with a little support or verbal mediation from me, he happily completed them, crying "more, more" after each one. As he cried "more," Ernie flapped his hands with excitement and rocked back and forth in the little chair.

A conventional view of Ernie's intense hand-flapping might have considered this flapping as a "clincher," proof positive that Ernie was autistic. While it is true that genuinely autistic children are prone to hand-flapping or other stereotypical behavior, the inverse—that all children who flap their hands are necessarily autistic—is not true. There are other developmental possibilities that might account for a child's hand flapping: excess tension, perhaps, or sensory overload. Consider, too, that virtually all infants at a certain stage of development flap their hands. For most this passes, as the child's nervous system and purposeful coordination mature. Some children, though, get stuck in this infant phase. Certainly the description by the foster father of Ernie's early years supported a hypothesis of lack of positive parental involvement, a factor that could account for him getting developmentally "stuck." It was clear that Ernie's hand flapping would require therapeutic work to help him regulate the powerful (hypothesized) combination of impoverished nurturance, tension and the force of habit.

It was also clear that Ernie was unquestionably joyful and excited about being challenged, about learning. His enthusiasm, his ability to learn from a model and to generalize his learning, his attention and concentration span—these were more than islets. They formed a continent! So although his eye contact was iffy at times, and although he did not engage in meaningful symbolic play, and although his language usage typified that of a very young toddler, on the other side of the ledger, the child that had been obscured by the symptoms was coming through loud and clear.

Ernie did not want to stop doing these challenging puzzles, but it was now four in the afternoon and our appointment was ending. Had I focused on his symptoms, I might have been tempted to conclude that Ernie, indeed, was highly impaired developmentally, even autistic, and that his special setting was appropriate for his needs. But the focus on his many islets of normalcy, above and beyond symptom presentation, indicated that here was a child with a wonderful capacity to grow, learn and change.

It was clear to me that my involvement with Ernie's progress was going to be long-term and would require active involvement and advocacy in facing a system which is symptom focused. His foster parents were no longer young and would be limited in their ability to interface with the educational system. But their everyday impressions of Ernie as an aware and intelligent child were correct. At the end of this first appointment I told them so.

Since the mandate of the Institute is not only to assess children and to offer treatment, but also to support and guide child and parents long-term through the odyssey of development, I made a series of appointments for Ernie in order to further assess his abilities, and asked for the foster parents' permission to observe Ernie in his special kindergarten. That visit proved to be a prelude to the dramatically challenging but ultimately successful process of having him transferred from his special setting to educational inclusion in a typical kindergarten with a gifted, devoted teacher.

I explained to his caregivers that we had a long but very worthwhile developmental journey ahead of us. I did not know then what lay ahead of us, which proved to be, in fact, a journey of many years of involvement and advocacy on Ernie's behalf—years that were laden with joy in seeing him progress, and then heartbreak when various support systems failed him as he approached puberty. There is no doubt, however, that Ernie's strong islets of normalcy—in particular his enthusiasm and delight in learning—helped to catapult him into a richer and more functional childhood than the specialist's report had ever predicted.

Sammy[2]

Sammy's first assessment appointment at the Institute was no less dramatic, and the unexpected emergence of islets of normalcy helped propel him as well to years of a more normalized childhood. Sammy was just three years old when he first came to the Institute. I had read the referral material which included a specialist's report from another setting, along with parallel reports from other medical and therapeutic practitioners on that team, all of whom had concurred that Sammy was autistic. Those practitioners had labeled him PDD (Pervasive Developmental Disorder), used at the time by most mental health and child development professionals as a synonym for an autistic condition.

His parents, whose energies had been sapped in raising Sammy's older sister who had special needs, described Sammy as not talking and not relating. They had only recently received the latest report from a specialist, and they were reeling from shock and smoldering grief that Sammy had been diagnosed as autistic (PDD).

Sammy was adorable. He reminded me of a cuddly roly-poly little teddy bear. He had a sturdy build and, I noted as he entered my office and just barely looked around the room, he had good motor coordination. There were no signs of dysmorphia (facial asymmetry) or other soft signs that might indicate a physiologically-based developmental problem. However, Sammy was clearly in deep developmental trouble.

He was not talking. He was effectively avoiding eye contact with his parents and with me. He did not approach his parents for comfort or connection. He wandered around my small office with no particularly apparent goal. I opened the toy cupboard. Sammy was interested. He began poking around, handling the sundry toys. I decided to limit the number of toys he could pull out of the cupboard. I selected a few, set them on the floor, and closed the cupboard door.

Sammy was not pleased. He exploded in rage. Like a whale that breeches the surface of the water and then slams its enormous bulk broadside on the waves, Sammy slammed himself onto the floor and began screaming. His parents looked distressed. The session did not look promising, and I was feeling a bit stymied by what appeared to be his resolute avoidance of contact and connection. While Sammy continued to tantrum, I tried to think of some musical, movement or play strategy that might "catch" Sammy and lure him into connection.

It was Sammy himself who solved the problem. When he had recovered from his tantrum (without having sought a soothing cuddle from his parents), Sammy suddenly began to push around my office furniture—the large chairs, the smaller chairs and the small table for children, and even my desk! Feeling a bit overwhelmed by the frustrating half hour that had preceded this, I stood behind my desk and just watched. Whatever was he doing? Sammy seemed to know. He continued to move the furniture until he had created a little row of chairs, big and small, which led to the summit—my desk top! He climbed onto the little chair at the beginning of the line of chairs he had arranged, and walked along them until he reached the top of my desk with a very pleased and proud look on his face.

Sammy spoke! Loudly! "One, two, three, jump!!" And he did, landing on the carpet between his equally surprised parents. He was not finished. He applauded himself, "Yay!!" And as he applauded, he looked directly at one parent and then the other, inviting them with his now expressive eye contact to applaud him and to share the experience.

Sammy had a wonderful time for the duration of this first assessment session. He continued climbing onto the row of chairs, reaching the top of my desk, jumping onto the carpet, then delightedly and with a huge warm smile applauding himself and "inviting" his parents to applaud and appreciate along with him. Sammy continued to count and say "jump" each time he leaped off my desk. Sometimes he counted in correct English and sometimes in correct Hebrew.

Once in a while, he made a little pit stop at the mirror hung at child level on my office wall. Before attempting his next climb, he would stand in front of the mirror, looking at himself with bright eyes and a warm smile of self-appreciation, while he spoke ample gibberish or jargon. Sammy was conducting a real gibberish conversation with himself as he looked in the mirror. As he did so, he gesticulated with wonderfully rich hand gestures, much as a lecturer might use to stress a point. As he delivered several gibberish "lectures" to himself, his tone of voice rose and fell with a kind of conscious musical rhythm that seemed to be indicating gibberish phrases and sentences, none of which were understandable. Sammy was very happy. So were his parents and so was I. Sammy's play proved to be a remarkable breakthrough, and a powerful display of rich and developmentally varied and significant islets of normalcy.

Sammy's initial presentation—of strongly avoidant eye contact, lack of emotional connection, combined with a lack of interpersonal communicative intent as well as speech—at first glance had signaled serious developmental impairment, and a strong candidacy for a diagnosis of PDD or autism, as the most recent specialist had concluded. But when Sammy recovered from his tantrum and began to initiate play in a way that was most meaningful to him, he displayed an enormous repertoire of islets of normalcy. In the ensuing discussion, I provide a "replay" of Sammy's behavior and elucidate the many islets that proved to be an exciting basis for our further work with him.

Returning to Sammy's foraging in the toy cupboard, in retrospect, we note that:

- Although not interested in the assessor, Sammy was interested in rummaging through the toys. This was an islet of normalcy—complete with intentionality, purposefulness, curiosity and exploratory behavior.
- His ensuing tantrum showed that Sammy was not indifferent to his surroundings. He had preferences, strong feelings and a strong will.
- Although he was not then speaking, he was certainly able to express frustration, loud and clear. His was not a flat, emotionless presentation.

In what could be considered inverse fashion, I noted that missing from Sammy's "autistic" presentation was any form of stereotypical behavior—hand flapping, rocking, spinning objects, walking in circuits. His "speaking with his hands" in front of the mirror was anything but stereotypical. He was pointing and gesticulating, with a delighted and amused expression in his eyes. He appeared to be imitating us adults who take ourselves so seriously when we talk.

- In short, Sammy's relaxed and purposeful body movements, without a trace of tense stereotypy, could be considered yet another islet of normalcy.
- Similarly, his delightful and uncanny use of hand gestures.

Most certainly, it was Sammy's energetic and purposeful play initiatives, arranging then jumping off my office furniture and all that then ensued, which yielded a large number of islets of normalcy:

- Sammy's arranging of the furniture was purposeful, goal-directed and meaningful.
- As he did this, he had a lovely excited smile on his face. This was not the rote activity of a child cut off from emotion. This was a normative play activity of an enthusiastic preschooler.
- Sammy's jumping off the table indicated that he had correctly assessed that this was a height he could manage. This indicated his attending and relating to at least some of the details of his surroundings.
- Sammy's counting was replete with islets of normalcy. Sammy revealed that he knew numbers and could count meaningfully in context, in English and in Hebrew. If he hadn't yet started speaking, as it had earlier appeared, he certainly had been attending to and absorbing at least the elements of two languages. How much more latent speech lay within him?
- His counting and then jumping reflected awareness of sequence and anticipation.
- Sammy's self-applauding was another lovely display of appropriate use of gestural communication.
- His attendant looks and smiles to each parent reflected the warmth he felt toward each, as well as a capacity for social referencing, as he invited them with warm eye contact and gestures (applause) to share his pleasure in accomplishment.

His pauses in front of the mirror were equally laden with islets of normalcy:

- The modulated intonations and rhythms of his gibberish were wonderful indications that Sammy possessed a normative prosody (the rhythmic underlying music and tonality unique to each language). Sammy's jargon, though indeed gibberish and undecipherable, really did sound like a spoken language. Sammy was not at all displaying the monotonic robot-like tones of a cut off and emotionless child.
- Sammy smiled and even laughed at himself as he lectured. He displayed a sense of humor—a wonderful islet necessary for emotional health.

- Sammy punctuated and exaggerated his gibberish speeches with a delightful range of hand motions, pointing, gesticulating and widening his eyes as his voice rose in a crescendo to make a point. He truly looked and sounded much like a little university professor making some very important points.

However, the most important point that Sammy was making was that, behind his initially worrisome presentation, there lay an emotionally vibrant child with the capacity for purposeful behavior and, most importantly, a capacity for interpersonal communication: gibberish, actual language, meaningful gestures, humor and enthusiasm and a range of normative emotions. These varied islets of normalcy provided a strong basis for our further work with Sammy over roughly the next four years, which saw Sammy transform from a child at risk to a child who could speak, learn to read and write and enjoy pretend play.

Islets as Developmental Leverage

Ernie and Sammy, like the hundreds and even thousands of young children whom my Institute colleagues and I assessed and worked with over the years, have much to teach us regarding the pitfalls of conventional diagnostic assessment on one hand and, on the other hand, the developmental leverage that the search for islets of normalcy gives us. During the assessment process and in the course of treatment, the focus on islets of normalcy—rather than on pathology or symptomatology—with children with suspected or confirmed autism provided a powerful launching pad for a much more promising developmental trajectory.

As Ernie and Sammy have illustrated, the symptoms, impairments, blocks, difficulties and developmental challenges of each child were all too obvious, even at first glance. Granted, it *is* important to note a child's symptoms—their description, their strength, their duration and frequency, certainly their prevalence in the child's profile. We do want to get a clear and detailed description of the condition in which a child first presents. However, we are not seeking a description of symptoms in order to clinch a diagnosis, a common practice in psychology today. We are seeking a description of the symptoms in order to help us strategize how best to change and modify the child's profile.

In order to do that, we must pay close attention not only to which symptoms are present and how often they appear, but more importantly, to the islets of normalcy, so that we can influence the malleability, the plasticity, the essential modifiability of the child's symptoms. A clinician working within the Feuerstein mindset is constantly asking him- or herself: "Can I as a clinician bring about change in the child's presentation, even in a marginal or microscopic way? If so, how to intervene?" Attending to islets of normalcy provides that springboard toward meaningful intervention.

During an initial session, as we take note of the child's difficulties, we must invest proportionally much more effort and energy to ascertain the child's strengths. Islets of normalcy, regardless of how faint, infrequent or microscopic they are, attest to the child's latent strengths. In a conventional method of assessing a child, the compilation of symptoms leads to a *diagnosis*. In the reciprocal, dynamic way of assessing and treating a child, the energetic interaction kindled by the therapist's initiatives and efforts to glean evidence of the latent health buried beneath the symptoms leads to an *understanding* of the child's functioning, to what Feuerstein called a profile of modifiability. To creatively mix metaphors, the islets of normalcy are like tiny sparks which we want to fan, through interactive play or creative cognitive intervention, so that they will grow to become a warm developmental blaze.

When we focus on the islets of normalcy during initial and ensuing sessions, the positive impact of this paradigm shift from symptom emphasis to normalcy emphasis is no less dramatic on the child's parents. As a rule, as I have noted throughout, parents of children elsewhere diagnosed, or suspected of falling into an autistic category, themselves would arrive at my office carrying a heavy emotional load. In previous encounters with other educational, developmental or medical practitioners, they had usually encountered a strict emphasis by the clinician on the child's symptom presentation, which had often resulted in a "confirmed diagnosis." Sometimes parents themselves had misgivings about their child's development and with great trepidation had researched on the internet extensive descriptions of "common symptoms" of autism, and without the input of any practitioners these parents had suspected, feared or concluded (often incorrectly) that their child suffered from autism.

The outlook of parents, who characteristically arrived at my office with an enormous load of pessimism and apprehension, usually brightened when they observed a different type of assessment, one which was playful and patient when encountering the child's symptoms and difficulties, one which was respectful of the child's choices, and above all, one in which the therapist enumerated for them during and at the end of the session the islets of normalcy which had been observed. Most parents visibly relaxed. Some wept with relief.

It is important, though, not only to identify and describe the islets of normalcy to parents but also to explain and even to teach parents the powerful developmental significance of islets of normalcy. I typically invested much time explaining to parents how these tiny strands of promising functioning can accrue and so gradually become strong cords of development. I further explained to parents how this emphasis on modifiability, the watchword of the Feuerstein perspective, and the focus on the identification of islets of normalcy can be used to inform a new vision of their child's prognosis.

I gave the parents positive "homework." To replace the parents' understandable hyperfocus on the symptoms of the child, I encouraged them to be on the lookout between appointments for their child's islets of normalcy. It was critical, at the end of each session, to give parents concrete tips and strategies to help them strengthen and enlarge islets of normalcy in their child's daily life. These tips often included, for example, clear guidelines for speaking amply and richly to even a nonverbal child, "soliloquy" in Feuerstein parlance, as well as helpful ideas for turning isolated behaviors into reciprocal ones, many of which were based on DIRFloortime strategies.

When Ernie and Sammy first arrived at the Institute, they were clearly in serious developmental trouble. A superficial observation of their presenting symptoms might easily have led to a confirmation of their previous diagnoses of autism and PDD respectively. Ernie appeared initially as communication- and cognitively-impaired. It would have been all too easy, using formalized criteria, to end that first session arriving at the diagnosis of autism, as other specialists had done. However, as the session wore on, and I moved from the phase of unfettered observation to active involvement with Ernie, islets of normalcy accrued. Ernie's cognitive functioning with increasingly difficult puzzles along with his overwhelming enthusiasm for relationship-supported learning and then his incipient speech tipped the balance of presumptions from "incapable" to "capable" to an exciting degree.

Similarly, at first glance Sammy appeared to be stubbornly avoiding eye contact and emotional contact, and there were no signs of intentionally in-teractive or symbolic play. Could it be other than an autistic type of diagnosis? Perhaps it was his explosive tantrum that helped him to release tension so that he then felt free to express a genuine interest in purposeful, active play. Perhaps he sensed a certain atmosphere of freedom and acceptance in my office that I would not object if he playfully rearranged the room. I hope so. Ultimately, it was his self-initiated play that revealed varied and impressive islets of normalcy: cognitive abilities, communicative abilities and emotional richness buried beneath his avoidant presentation. Using these islets of nor-malcy as our basis for understanding his latent abilities, I accompanied Sammy for many years on his developmental journey as he went on to enjoy normative speech capabilities, the ability to engage in humor-laden and imaginative symbolic play, and the acquisition of reading, writing and basic math skills.

Later in their educational careers, Ernie and Sammy each encountered unfortunate administrative barriers within the educational system and/or experienced emotional/situational crises, whose combination left their young adulthoods less than happy. Despite this fact, I have selected Ernie and Sammy as prime examples of the impact of the clinical focus on islets of normalcy, because their initial sessions were highly dramatic, with a clear and powerful distinction between superficial symptom presentation and their fine latent developmental abilities evidenced in their islets of normalcy. There is no doubt that the focus on islets of normalcy as a basis for dynamic assessment and ensuing treatment resulted in years of happier and more productive childhoods for each child.

Ernie and Sammy were not alone. Using the positive outlook of searching for islets of normalcy so central to the Feuerstein philosophy, and en-ergetically creating islets even when they were not yet evident, my colleagues and I had the great satisfaction of watching many children, who arrived at the Institute having been diagnosed as autistic, PDD or ASD, continue on a path in which our team supported and guided them to near-normative and even normative functioning in the realms of verbal communication, peer relationships and learning.

Notes

1 This chapter, for which the author holds copyright, first appeared under the same title in *Feuerstein on Autism*, edited by Rafael S. Feuerstein, and published in 2019 by the Feuerstein Institute in Jerusalem. It appeared on pages 68 through 87.
2 A different version of Sammy's story appeared as a chapter by the author entitled "Barriers, Bridges, Breakthroughs: Play Work with Autistic Spectrum Children" on pages 77 through 110 in *The International Handbook of Play Therapy: Advances in Assessment, Theory, Research, and Practice*, edited by Charles Schaefer, Judy McCormick, and Akiko Ohnogi, and published in 2005 by Jason Aronson of New York. Parts of that chapter have been revised and are reprinted herein with permission.

References

Levin, Shoshana. "Barriers, Bridges, Breakthroughs: Play Work with Autistic Spectrum Children." In *The International Handbook of Play Therapy: Advances in Assessment, Theory, Research, and Practice*, edited by Charles Schaefer, Judy McCormick, and Akiko Ohnogi, 77–110. New York: Jason Aronson, 2005.

Levin Fox, Shoshana. "Searching for Islets of Normalcy." In *Feuerstein on Autism*, edited by Rafael S. Feuerstein, 68–87. Jerusalem: Feuerstein Institute, 2019.

11 DIRFloortime Basics

Playing with a young child is always enjoyable. But playing with a young child experiencing developmental challenges in a way that yields developmental benefits is a delight. It was within the realm of play—whether sensory-based baby playtime, kinesthetic (active, motor) or imaginative and symbolic—that the developmental progress for nearly all of the children in this book was jumpstarted. Although play is not part and parcel of the Feuerstein method, play is pivotal in reaching young children. In the late 1990s and following, Professor Feuerstein took a nucleus of his staff to the United States to attend several major conferences on autism organized by Drs. Stanley Greenspan and Serena Wieder, under the auspices of the Interdisciplinary Council on Development and Learning (ICDL).[1] Following these conferences and some continued training in Floortime, when using Feuerstein methods and theories to assess and treat young children with autistiform symptoms, I began to interweave the developmental wisdom and progressive play strategies of DIRFloortime within the dynamic assessment work. It was wonderful to discover that, though very different in conceptualization and content from Feuerstein's theories, DIR methods worked comfortably within the Feuerstein context.

This chapter relays the essential outline of the DIR stages and strategies, which proved to be playfully useful in dynamically assessing and treating autistiform children. The DIR stages and strategies coupled with the philosophic outlook of Feuerstein's vision related to human modifiability proved to be a potent, effective and enjoyable combination for working creatively and effectively with these children. Since I had already learned to speak the language of play with young children in my play therapy training, it was a comfortable hop into the world of Floortime.

Developed by the late child psychiatrist Stanley Greenspan and clinical psychologist Serena Wieder, DIRFloortime is a form of therapist-coached and parent-powered interactive developmental intervention. The graphic term Floortime helps emphasize the focus and realm of activity, particularly in the early stages: on the floor with the child and playfully attuned to the child's presenting state. The initials DIR signify a developmental approach (D), sensitive to individual differences (I), and relationship based (R). Greenspan and Wieder have elucidated their theory and its practical applications in numerous sources.[2,3,4] This chapter summarizes the essentials of that approach which is used widely, though not solely, with children with autistiform symptoms. DIR strategies, with their developmental play emphasis, proved to be an effective complement to the Institute's focus on dynamic (qualitative, functionally descriptive, interactive) assessment and intervention in working with children who presented with autistic features.

Roots

Experts in the field of infant neurodevelopment and child development, Greenspan and Wieder, during their early collaborative years, researched normative infant development in a relational context between mothers and young children at the National Institute of Mental Health. Their cumulative work led to an in-depth understanding of the mother-child relationship, and more pertinently, enabled them to develop teachable interactive mother-child communication strategies to help parents build the critical initial rapport and emotional basis necessary for the child's further development.[5] Ultimately, they identified six social emotional stages of early childhood development. Three additional stages pertaining to more advanced, nuanced and flexible thinking were later added to the original model.[6] They further identified a set of functional developmental goals or milestones relevant to each stage that the child needs to achieve in order to successfully negotiate progress to the next stage. Full mastery of each of these stages and their milestones is the goal of DIR interventions. There is a dynamic overlap among the stages with an overall progressive developmental direction.

There is clear and cogent vision in this theoretical roadmap for the child's climbing the developmental ladder. A child who successfully achieves the developmental goals of these successive stages should be an aware, communicative, relating, playful child who can learn from and respond to the environment through emotional investment, increasingly rich language and symbolic play. Later, that child can advance to achieve more emotionally complex symbolic play, emotional/social problem solving, and conceptual and abstract thinking. The parent, caregiver or clinician is always watchful to ensure that even the child who appears to be functioning in accord with the latter stages of the model has thoroughly met the milestones of the earlier stages.

In their work which served as a precursor to the development of DIR, Greenspan and Wieder focused on empowering parents whose relational skills were weak or even impaired, by teaching and coaching them to carry out their recommended practical play-based interventions to enhance parent-child relationship and communication. The children began to change as parents became more skillful at interacting and communicating. The parents became more confident. The work of Greenspan and Wieder yielded positive results even among children whose developmental profiles were challenging and complex and/or whose parents initially lacked the skills and the confidence to assist their children.[7]

Greenspan and Wieder realized that the developmental ladder which they envisioned, with its particular stages and related goals, contained developmental power. Genuinely autistic children do not relate, often leading to frustration, pain and discouragement in their parents. These clinicians asked themselves a powerful question: what would happen if parents of autistic children were trained and coached to envision the same developmental goals and to negotiate the same developmental stages in the naturally playful and attuned manner that had been shown to be effective with children with other developmental challenges? Hence the birth of the DIRFloortime paradigm for autistic children with its developmentally sensitive six stages.

The Six Developmental Stages and Their Milestones

Self-Regulation and Interest in the World[8]

In Stage One, Self-Regulation and Interest in the World, the infant or young child must be able to recover from a state of excitement, overstimulation or distress and return to a state of calm. Conversely, in this stage, the child should be able to sustain initial interest in the world without becoming overly stimulated and overwhelmed on one hand and without lapsing into prolonged avoidance or withdrawal on the other. An overly excited or distressed child who is unable to calm will not be accessible to connection and relationship. A withdrawn or apathetic infant or child will need to be energized to become more aware of the world.

Drawing from the sensory integration literature in the field of occupational therapy, notably the work of Ayres,[9] Greenspan and Wieder weighted their understanding of infant and early childhood regulation toward attuning to children's patterns of sensory reactivity. Is the infant or young autistiform child hyporeactive or hyposensitive to various sounds, colors, textures, movements? Is the child hyper-reactive or hypersensitive to such stimuli? Or is the child's sensory profile a complex mix, hyposensitive to some stimuli, hypersensitive to others? The child who screams because of the blender's whirring may be hypersensitive to auditory stimuli. An infant's gazing at the ceiling for hours might reflect an under-reactive profile. Each child and adult has his or her own sensory diet of sensory stimuli that arouse or irritate, calm or soothe.

In this model, particularly in the early stages, the parent's attunement to an infant's or autistiform child's sensory preferences and degree of reactivity can impact strongly on the process of development. The parent's or the practitioner's initial goal, then, is to attune to the child's degree of sensitivity and reactivity and playfully bring the child to a capacity for self-regulation. For example, a hyposensitive and hyporeactive baby lying passively in a crib for hours needs the input and stimulation of active parental strategies (for example, by tickling or rocking the child or by using stimulating auditory or visual play materials).

By this model, the mother who is calm and quiet herself would need to learn active strategies to help her baby energize, using sensory and motor play so that the infant moves from apathy toward displaying more active interest in the world. Similarly, a highly sensitive and reactive infant or young child, screaming at each new sound, movement or texture, will require parental play and communication strategies that convey soothing and calming (gentle rocking, singing softly) so that he or she can begin to interact comfortably in the world.

Play strategies associated with this first stage emerge from this sensitive attunement to the autistiform child's sensory profile and degree of reactivity. Play activities that can be called "baby playtime" (rocking, singing, gentle tickling) are not just for babies. As Greenspan and Wieder advocate, the adaptation of attuned early infant relationship strategies with children who present with autistiform features creates a necessary and positive basis for later development. Allowing "regression" to these levels, and playfully indulging early regulatory needs, is actually not regression at all but rather part of a process which builds the basis for and yields pathways to further meaningful developmental progress.

Engagement, Attachment and Intimacy

The child who is no longer caught at the extremes of being too overwhelmed or too avoidant—that is, who is now capable of self-regulation—is then able to progress to Stage Two, with the milestone of a sense of Engagement, Attachment and Intimacy. The child is now accessible enough, neither overwhelmed nor apathetic, to respond to the adult's overtures for contact with signs of pleasure.

In this stage, even before language emerges, the young child is learning about the primary emotional reality of warmth in a nonverbal dialogue of emotional reciprocity. Warm eye contact, little smiles, pleasure in receiving comforting touch, distress when warm contact is interrupted—all indicate that the young child is learning the basic language of emotional interest, intimacy and pleasurable connection.

The DIRFloortime strategies associated with this stage stress creating an atmosphere of warmth and pleasure in contact. The adult is not directing, but following the child's lead and joining him or her in simple activities that reach the child and which can be used to elicit pleasure in contact and shared attention. Humorous engagement with the child, pleasurable baby playtime, tickles, simple sensory and movement activities—all these and more are employed to woo the child toward experiences of openness to, and delight in, warm contact. The medium is the message. It is fun and pleasurable to be in contact, to be together.

Intentional Two-Way Communication

Building on this ability to delight in and share emotional energy, in Stage Three the toddler or young child begins to show signs of being able to engage in simple Intentional Two-Way Communication. This level of communication is largely, though not solely, nonverbal.

Within the DIR paradigm, the term "circles of communication" is the essential unit of meaningful interactive communication. Very rudimentary circles of communication can begin to appear even in the stage of Intimacy. The baby smiles (opening a circle of communication) and mother smiles back (closing the circle). Mother then sings to baby (opening another circle), and baby smiles and coos with pleasure (closing another circle) and waving her arms (opening another circle to which the mother can respond). A child who has begun to enjoy warm attachment may exhibit displeasure or distress when the adult is unavailable. In such a case, the distress itself serves as part of a circle of communication, a positive sign that rudimentary attachment is evolving.

This third stage of Intentional Two-Way communication, with its opening and closing of a gradually increasing number of circles of nonverbal communication (eye contact, gestures), ultimately lays the foundation for speech. An infant engages in two-way communication when he or she imitates a parent's cooing sounds or shares meaningful eye contact in a peek-a-boo game. The young child engages in two-way communication even through the simplest of nonverbal gestures: he or she reaches out to be picked up, or takes mother's hand to open the door. The dialogue of intimacy through amorphous feelings begins to assume a more tangible form in intentional gestures, imitative movements, imitative vocalization (babbling), first words and nuance-laden eye contact in response to the situation.

To build early circles of communication, Greenspan and Wieder advised that adults always position themselves facing the child, follow the child's play lead and actively join in to create more circles. Sometimes, DIR recommends that doing the unexpected, even the playfully provocative, can lead to a sense of emotional contact. The adult can be proactive and initiate play ideas, for example, joining an avoidant child in lining up his cars, accepting the child's frustrated anger as part of a circle of communication, waiting a few seconds and then adding another car to his line. Or, as a child points in frustration to a toy she cannot reach on the shelf, the adult working in this model may choose to "play dumb," upping the emotional valence and provoking the child into even more insistent expression and contact. Even angry annoyance on the part of the child is a form of contact and communicative response, which the adult can then reflect and use to gently move up the developmental ladder: "You really want that toy and you're upset. Shall I hand you this one or that one?" The DIR paradigm reminds the practitioner that even dissonance and frustration can be used, with utmost caution and sensitivity of course, to woo the child into further circles of communication and emotional relationship. The overall goal of this and the following stages is to create increasingly long chains of circles of communication. The parent's ability to respond to and participate in these preverbal exchanges thus strengthens the child and lays the foundation for Stage Four, with its milestone of achieving Complex Communication.

Complex Communication

In Stage Four, Complex Communication, the child can respond purposefully with a series or combination of gestures, vocalization and even words to achieve a desired relationship or communication goal. Both the number and the quality of the circles of communication are increasing. The child remains communicative through words, touch, gestures, play activity or an increasingly complex combination of these in a relational context. The developmental emphasis in this stage is the chaining of various elements of communication: the child whimpers, looks at mother, walks over to her, pulls her hand toward the shopping bag, urges her to take out a bag of chips, and says "Candy, mmmm." Here the child has successfully chained several preverbal and verbal communicative components, circles of communication, to achieve a goal within a relational context.

In a play context, the adult is responding to the child's lead with the aim of keeping the play interaction going and expanding it, using a range of play activities still attuned to the child's sensory preferences and level of regulatory abilities. This could be a game of hide and seek, tossing a ball back and forth or using interesting cause-and-effect toys to pique interest and involvement. At a more advanced developmental level, activities at this stage can include simple symbolic play. The adult is not only thinking of the goals of self-regulation, shared pleasure and communication, nonverbal and verbal, but is also gradually moving toward more complex pretend play activities, while sometimes even gently challenging the child in order to keep the circles of communication going. Beyond the realm of immediate needs, the young child is now able to express communicative intent through an increasingly varied repertoire of gestures, vocalization and even words to express personal states, wants and needs. The child can respond to the adult's collaborative play ideas or even initiate simple play activities.

Emotional Ideas

As Complex Communication skills evolve and accrue, the young child approaches DIR developmental Stage Five, expressing Emotional Ideas. Comfort with the world of simple pretend and symbolic play grows. The DIR term Emotional Ideas to a large extent parallels the common understanding of symbolic play. The child can now begin to collaborate with the adult or even initiate symbolic play ideas, such as feeding dolly or putting her to sleep. The child's repertoire of symbolic expression modalities may include play, pictures and/or spoken language, as each of these realms has begun to assume meaning and expressive value for the child. The adult strives to expand the child's use of and comfort with an ever-widening range of emotional themes. Over the course of these developmental phases, the number of circles of communication which a child can open and close is continually increasing.

Emotional Thinking

Stage Six, Emotional Thinking, emphasizes the development of thought processes and the logical chaining of ideas which begin to enter the child's play. Symbolic play ideas are not isolated. They are beginning to be connected through logical understanding and a sense of logical sequence, such as: "First dolly wakes up, then she goes to the park." Cause and effect connections appear in the child's play and speech: "Bad dolly gets a spanking and no dinner. Next time no spilling." Or: "The doctor put grandma in the hospital because she was sick." Or even: "Sad raining."

The child's symbolic play is encouraged to become more elaborate, with the adult always seeking opportunities to raise and expand the developmental level of the play. This can mean, for example, the adult's asking questions to link symbolic play ideas with more sophisticated thinking about concepts and processes: "I see. We're taking our teddy bears to the store, but oh no! The store is closed now! What should we do?" Questions and additions to the child's play challenge the child to think, to process and to experience the fact that symbolic ideas are meaningful and can be expanded in their details. Whereas in Stage Three, Simple Two-Way Communication, the child's practical problem-solving was exciting evidence of progress (for example, the child's searching for the tiny car in the adult's pocket), by Stage Six problem solving is carried out in the increasingly complex spheres of emotional/social themes and symbolic play. At this stage, through play the child is doing increasingly more emotional, ideational and verbal processing.

Improved language, the ability to reason and the ability to solve practical and emotional challenges that arise within play, along with the ability to express these through a varied repertoire of symbolic behaviors, have emerged via a process of increasingly intricate emotional and communicative reciprocity. Precisely because the child has traversed a developmental path rich in affect and relationships that led from Self-Regulation, to Intimacy, to Intentional Simple then Complex Communication, to Emotional Ideas and Emotional Thinking, at this stage the young child, including the child who initially presented with autistiform symptoms, is now poised to move forward, to engage in cognitive tasks that involve reasoning, the processing of ideas and engaging in more formalized learning.

Following their basic configuration of this model, creators Greenspan and Wieder later added three more developmental stages to reflect the child's progression from increasingly complex and coherent symbolic play and expression into the world of Multi-Causal Thinking (Stage Seven), Emotionally Differentiated Thinking (Stage Eight) and Reflective Thinking and a Stable Sense of Self (Stage Nine). These latter stages, as elaborated in their 2006 book *Engaging Autism*, were less pertinent to the developmental levels of the predominantly young children whose stories are told in this book, as these children needed first to master the earlier stages of social communication development.

Greenspan and Wieder maintained that these six foundational stages and their associated milestones of normative child development can be understood and utilized as a developmental blueprint to be achieved by the child with social communication impairments. The entire thrust of DIR intervention, then, is to help parents and practitioners proactively employ specialized play techniques that have the power to move the child up the developmental ladder from a state of regulated attention to the world, to pleasurable engagement in a milieu of warmth and intimacy, to two-way communication that is at first nonverbal and then verbal and increasingly complex, to coaxing the child into pretend play skills and comfort with the expression of ideas and finally, toward helping the child develop notions of social/emotional problem-solving and patterns of more logical thinking as play becomes more meaningful, expressive and complex.

Parents Are Pivotal

The DIR developmental model views parents as pivotal to the development of a child with autistiform symptoms. In Floortime, parents are coached to use creative play techniques that attune to the child's developmental stage and sensory needs and then to work toward achievement of the identified milestones. Parents learn nonverbal and preverbal play strategies so that they can playfully build reciprocal communication with children in whom reciprocity at first appears to be entirely lacking. As the child with autistiform symptoms begins to engage, parents are coached to expand the child's functionally expressive repertoire, and ultimately, to expand the child's rudimentary verbal and symbolic play ideas.

Floortime strategies are creative and can be adapted to address certain challenging behaviors often typical of children who present as autistic. For example, a child's perseverative door-banging, instead of being considered annoying evidence of developmental pathology, becomes reframed in this paradigm as a potential opening for communication by the responsive adult. How to close such a circle? Greenspan and Wieder suggest, for example, that the adult get behind the door and turn the perseverative activity into meaningful interaction, perhaps by making each closure part of a peek-a-boo game. Or, a parent might playfully apply pressure to the door so that the child will even more actively try to close it, creating a nonverbal dialogue of action between parent and child. As noted, even a communication-challenged child's protest can be seen as an expression of meaningful contact with the world, with the child's every expression of anger offering another opportunity for an adult's communicative response.

A play-oriented attitude and play activities are intrinsic to every stage of DIR intervention. In the early developmental levels of this model, the play strategies are particularly attuned to sensory aspects, including movement, touch, and light or deep pressure (such as holding, rocking, swinging or tickling the child). The parents of a screaming child overwhelmed by the sound of the vacuum cleaner may learn to hold or rock the child gently while softly humming to achieve calm. Or, parents may be coached to avoid sensory input that is overwhelming or painful to the child until the child's sensory reactions are better regulated. Parents might opt to vacuum while the child is with grandma at the park!

As the child develops and improves, there are increasingly sophisticated play-based strategies to help the child move toward relationship. For example, if a child routinely lines up small cars in a row without averting his or her gaze from them, parents may be coached to playfully hoard the rest of the cars and tuck them one at a time into pockets. This playful maneuver forces the child into a circle of communication, perhaps digging into Dad's pocket or looking into Dad's eyes with an expressive whine.

In the higher developmental stages, parents are coached to add verbal strategies to their play repertoire, creating little problems for the child to solve, introducing new ideas, challenging the child and playfully encouraging the child to link ideas in a play context. Mother: "But dolly doesn't want to go to sleep. She's still very hungry and upset. How can we help her?" The creators of this paradigm encouraged parents to carry out DIRFloortime strategies as part of the child's everyday life in order to achieve maximum benefit, under the guidance of a professional trained in the method.

DIRFloortime Applied

The stories of the children in this casebook are replete with examples of playful Floortime strategies. I borrowed many of these strategies from DIR literature and training. Other play strategies were created in impromptu fashion to suit the needs and challenges of a given child at a given moment. Within the case story chapters, I opted not to specify the DIR stages that were applicable to each child. However, those stages and their milestones were often in my thoughts during the challenging work. A few examples: Gently tickling his feet helped Sasha (Chapter 2) to look up from his closed off world and glance at me. Annie (Chapter 3) began to calm, to appear less anxious and to relinquish a little eye contact when she cuddled up in the U-shaped swing and rocked. The developmental needs of these two children were generally typical of Stage One, Self-Regulation and Interest in the World. A sensory-based game helped Gordie (Chapter 12) share eye contact and warm toward a sense of Intimacy (Stage Two). Amy (Chapter 12) responded to a movement sequence activity that encouraged eye contact and the opening and closing of nonverbal circles of communication, suggesting that she was capable of Stage Three, Simple Intentional Two-Way Communication. Josh (Chapter 8) tentatively created a symbolic scene of a birthday party in the doll house, as he eyed me cautiously and whispered "birthday party." He used eye contact, language and rudimentary symbolic play to communicate, placing him in Stage Four of Complex Communication, with elements of later more symbolic stages embedded. Davie (Chapter 4) loved sitting at the table, working comfortably with the assessor and carrying out play-based preschool learning tasks that included story books. He responded to the stories with symbolic comprehension and interest, as characteristic of Stage Five, Emotional Ideas. Given Jack's interest in the personalities and worlds of his transformers, it was immediately evident that Jack (Chapter 1) arrived already functioning comfortably in the world of symbolic play, and could initiate logical play scenarios. He was exhibiting the Emotional Thinking characteristic of Stage Six.

The Richness of Two Worlds

The theories of Greenspan and Wieder emerged from the field of infant mental health, while the theories and methods of Feuerstein emerged from the sphere of cognitive psychology. DIR is a therapeutic method in its own right and is not part of the methodology of the Feuerstein Institute, and vice versa. The application of the developmentally sensitive DIRFloortime play strategies within the context of Feuerstein's emphasis on modifiability yielded an effective, synergistic assessment and treatment combination. The Institute, with its philosophy of and commitment to developing the maximum potential of the individual, provided fertile ground for my application of DIR strategies with children who presented with autistic symptoms during both dynamic assessment and subsequent treatment phases.

There were compatible points of theoretical and practical overlap between the world of Floortime and the world of Feuerstein. Feuerstein's emphasis on the focused intentionality of the mediator in eliciting a child's strengths echoed warmly in my mind with the Floortime concepts of actively entering the autistic-like child's play sphere, wooing the child and pursuing a sense of engagement. Feuerstein's notion of reciprocity, an energetic give-and-take, a flow of communication exchange between adult mediator and child learner, seemed to dovetail comfortably with the reciprocity inherent in the Floortime notion of creating circles of communication. Floortime prized the flashes of emergent contact, pleasure, shared attention, symbolic play, and therefore urged practitioners to expand these moments. In parallel, Feuerstein taught and demonstrated the power of seeking non-symptomatic behavior (islets of normalcy), prizing its significance and using it as a springboard for what, in many cases, launched a veritable developmental makeover.

And so, from the Floortime paradigm, I embraced the concept of the developmental ladder with its associated stages and strategies, and the notion of circles of communication. The idea of opening and closing circles of communication proved to be the driving mechanism I was using, while keeping in mind a kind of developmental mantra: "Keep looking for opportunities to open or close circles of communication! Keep looking for ways to expand the contact, chain these circles and keep this communicative energy going."

In parallel, when looking at each child through the lens of Feuerstein, that of potential modifiability, even the most miniscule examples of normative functioning, communication and relating mattered. If opening, closing and chaining circles of communication formed the energetic mechanism of work with even the most challenged children, Feuerstein's concept of islets of normalcy helped me locate within the sea of the child's symptoms some solid ground on which to begin that energetic work. The concept of islets of normalcy proved to be a mainstay in my work of dynamic assessment and intervention with young autistic-featured children, as the previous chapter introduced and the following chapter explores in greater detail, showing how these two distinct methods could be used in tandem.

Notes

1 The Interdisciplinary Council on Development and Learning is the not-for-profit organization founded by Stanley Greenspan to promote and teach DIRFloortime and the developmental model on which it is based.
2 Stanley I. Greenspan, *Infancy and Early Childhood: The Practice of Clinical Assessment and Intervention with Emotional and Developmental Challenges* (Madison, CT: International Universities Press, 1992).
3 Stanley I. Greenspan and Serena Wieder, *The Child with Special Needs: Encouraging Intellectual and Emotional Growth* (Reading, MA: Addison-Wesley, 1998).
4 Stanley I. Greenspan and Serena Wieder, *Engaging Autism: Using the Floortime Approach to Help Children Relate, Communicate and Think* (Boston, MA: DaCapo Press, 2006).
5 Serena Wieder, personal communication to the author on January 10, 2020, confirming presentation at Bar Ilan University training workshop; date untraceable.
6 Greenspan and Wieder, *Engaging Autism*.
7 Serena Wieder, personal communication to the author on January 10, 2020, confirming presentation at Bar Ilan University training workshop; date untraceable.
8 The DIR model is a dynamic one that continues to develop. As such, the reader may have encountered these stages captioned differently from the ones I have used. This is so, because the various stages are sometimes referred to differently in the literature, depending upon the reference source and its date. The general progressive developmental content and direction remain the same.
9 Anna Jean Ayres, "Characteristics of Types of Sensory Integrative Dysfunction," *American Journal of Occupational Therapy* 25 (1971): 329–34.

References

Ayres, Anna Jean. "Characteristics of Types of Sensory Integrative Dysfunction." *American Journal of Occupational Therapy* 25 (1971): 329–34.
Greenspan, Stanley I. *Infancy and Early Childhood: The Practice of Clinical Assessment and Intervention with Emotional and Developmental Challenges*. Madison, CT: International Universities Press, 1992.
Greenspan, Stanley I. and Serena Wieder. *The Child with Special Needs: Encouraging Intellectual and Emotional Growth*. Reading, MA: Addison-Wesley, 1998.
Greenspan, Stanley I. and Serena Wieder. *Engaging Autism: Using the Floortime Approach to Help Children Relate, Communicate and Think*. Boston, MA: DaCapo Press, 2006.

12 Islets of Normalcy Revisited

The stories of Ernie, Sammy and the other children in this book have much to teach us about the clinical power of searching for islets of normalcy. Parents and practitioners seeking to help a child with autistiform symptoms in a dynamic—interactive, qualitative, process- and change-focused—mode rather than a structured norm-based and symptom-focused conventional mode will need virtual binoculars and a virtual microscope to identify these islets. The binoculars metaphor signals that we are searching a vast overall behavioral and communication landscape for significant details, those islets which we want to strengthen and enlarge. The microscope metaphor reminds us that, especially in the early phases of the work, we will most likely not be dealing with clear and obvious evidence of normalcy. We will be seeking even the smallest islets of normative behavior.

In explaining to parents the concept of islets of normalcy, I sometimes switch metaphors and ask them whether they have ever lit a campfire. When they look puzzled, I explain that we are looking for the tiniest sparks of normative behavior or "anti-symptom" which we hope to gently fan into a warming developmental flame. To accomplish that, I have found that work which is grounded in the Feuerstein positive belief in human modifiability—focused on the search for islets of normalcy—and which is enriched by Floortime developmental play techniques can be quite effective.

How do we recognize an islet of normalcy? The islets of normalcy we are seeking pertain to a large range of developmental details: eye contact that is increasingly sustained, eye contact that is increasingly warm and relational, a sense of reciprocity, turn-taking abilities, interest in relationship, pleasure in contact and relationship, warmth, humor, curiosity, exploratory behavior, gestural communication, vocalization, babbling, vocal imitation, early speech and language, purposeful object use, symbolic play, expression of emotion, task orientation—and many more. When we identify these islets, no matter how fleeting, infrequent, weak or overshadowed by apparent symptoms in the child's profile, they are always significant. Once identified, islets become our basis and focus for intervention. If we have noted the activities that elicit these islets, and the interpersonal circumstances that nurture them, these very activities become the recommended avenues for continuing to treat the child in a relational context. Over time in this manner of working, the proportion of normative islets to symptomatic behaviors improves, and the impact of impairments, deficits or even pathology weakens as the child's strengths grow.

The notion of islets of normalcy helps both parent and practitioner recognize the non-symptomatic behavior, the sparks of life and the glimmers of normative functioning within a child's autistiform presentation. Paying attention over time to a child's developing islets of normalcy helps one gauge the scope of qualitative changes in the child's presentation: is normative functioning gradually increasing in proportion to the child's problematic functioning?

The Feuerstein term islets of normalcy and the DIR concept of circles of communication are not identical in theoretical formulation, but in practice, as noted, they proved to be complementary and the two concepts worked synergistically. The term "circles of communication" served as a vivid reminder of the energetic mechanism of desired communication on which the adult should be focused: keeping the sense of contact, shared attention, relationship and communication going. What was I looking for? Islets of normalcy. What should I try to do with them? Help the child open and close the circles of communication associated with each islet, and strive to chain together an increasingly large number of circles. And a further question: how and where to find these islets? The Floortime sensory pathways provide direction.

As described in Chapter 11, Greenspan and Wieder made a revolutionary contribution to the treatment of suspected and confirmed autism by describing clear functional developmental stages, and by enumerating many energetic, interactive play and communication strategies to help the child reach each given stage. Their DIRFloortime model derives particular power from the originators' identification of sensory modalities—sight, hearing, touch, movement—as key pathways to interpreting and to treating autistiform behavior. Acknowledging the work of Jean Ayres on sensory processing,[1] Greenspan and Wieder remind parents and practitioners to pay careful attention to each child's unique sensory profile, whether hyposensitive, hypersensitive or mixed.

From the perspective of Feuerstein's dynamic, interactive mode of assessing and treating suspected autism, tallying numbers of symptoms does not even begin to help us understand the particularities of a child's social communication difficulty. There are so many nuances and gradations of the child's symptoms and strengths (those precious islets again) to which one must attend. Fast forward to the sensory attunement of the DIRFloortime model which alerts us that each sensory modality permits welcome new opportunities for sensitively opening and closing circles of communication. These same sensory channels, I found, similarly provide opportunities for identifying, developing and creating islets of normalcy even when at first they do not exist.

As the DIRFloortime model teaches, the sensory channels of vision, hearing, touch and movement serve as points of entry to understanding and working productively with a child who is thought to be autistic. To that end, the Floortime originators suggested questions intended to help parents and practitioners attune to each child's unique sensory differences. Within the

Floortime paradigm, the answers to these sensory-focused questions provide points of departure for opening and closing circles of communication with the child. From the Feuerstein perspective, the answers to these same functional questions help one reach a differential understanding of where and how previously obscured strengths and islets of normalcy can be found or elicited.

And so, when seeing a child with autistic features, my mind is always firing with dozens of qualitative, functional questions about what I am observing and its relevance as I interact with the child using play or learning materials. When observing and playfully interacting with a child, the practitioner working dynamically will be asking him- or herself many qualitative questions, some of which are interrelated, that is, pertaining to the interplay of the various sensory channels. Questions in the following text are borrowed from, adapted from or inspired by DIRFloortime sources.[2]

The Visual Channel

We want to know much more than whether the child's eye contact is avoidant or engaging, because a simple "yes" or "no" answer will not take us far in identifying and engaging a child's latent strengths. We want to know:

- Under what circumstances is the child's eye contact engaged?
- Under what circumstances is the child's eye contact avoidant?
- What sensory, motor or other play activities help the child gradually restore eye contact or reduce avoidance?
- What sensory channels and activities encourage more engaged eye contact? Does the child's eye contact improve if the adult softly sings to the child? Plays with or holds the child in front of the mirror? Gently rocks the child? Gently tickles the child? Helps the child to jump?
- What sensory situations and activities that inhibit eye contact need to be minimized? The adult's loud voice? Other loud noises? The adult moving too closely or too quickly into the child's space? Touch that is too firm?
- Does the quality of the child's eye contact change from avoidant to engaging or vice versa according to contexts (for example, improve in a larger or a quieter play space)?
- Does the quality of the child's eye contact differ according to persons (for example, more engaged with grandma than with mother)?
- When the child does make eye contact, what emotions are reflected in his or her eyes? Fear? Anger? Indifference? Warmth? Surprise? Love? Delight?
- How does the duration of the child's eye contact vary within and across interpersonal and sensory contexts?
- When and in what interpersonal or sensory situations is the child's eye contact more sustained and relational? When is eye contact fleeting? What is the impact of other sensory channels on the duration of a child's eye contact? More sustained when being gently held? More sustained when there are no extraneous noises?

- Does the quality of the child's eye contact change in relation to his or her distance from the adult? Is eye contact better if the adult is further from the child?
- What changes in the child's eye contact occur if the adult pretends not to notice the child, or actively avoids the child's eyes in order to reduce any sense of threat?
- Which visual stimuli calm and focus the child? Attract the child? Colorful objects? Moving objects, such as a ball? Bright objects, such as shiny gold cloth?
- Which visual stimuli entice the child into contact?
- Bubbles! Do the child's eye contact and relational openness improve when the adult creates a screen of bubbles that eases the potential threat of direct visual contact?

The Auditory Channel

Before exploring the auditory channel in the search to find or elicit islets of normalcy, the clinician will first want to ascertain some basic facts about the child's auditory history that have serious consequences for the path of language acquisition and important implications as to whether the child may be genuinely autistic or not:

- Does the child have a documented hearing loss? At what age was this loss discovered? What interventions were carried out following the discovery?
- Is there a history of hyperacute hearing? Children with hypersensitive hearing, for whom loud noises are literally painful, may have "turned off" their hearing in order to avoid discomfort. Many of these children may prove not to be autistic at all.
- Is there a history of chronic ear infections and fluids? As noted in an earlier chapter, while there are children with a history of ear fluids who are genuinely autistic, there are many children with chronic ear infections and fluids who experience an expressive language delay, and who are then mistakenly diagnosed as autistic.

Fine-tuning our attention to nuances of the child's auditory sensitivity, we will then want to note:

- How do the adult's vocal tone, pitch and rhythm of speech affect the sense of engagement with the child? How do variations in these affect the child's eye contact? For example, is a soft wooing tone of voice or a rhythmic clipped tone of voice more likely to elicit islets of normalcy, such as a responsive smile?
- How do changes in the adult's vocal pitch, tone or rhythm of speech affect the child's attentional/relational/emotional state? Does the child become calmer with a certain tone of voice or more agitated?

- What are the effects of musical stimuli, such as musical toys or background music, on the child's sense of connectedness, relatedness, engagement and awareness of others?
- What are the effects of auditory stimuli in creating a sense of connection with the child? Does the child move closer when addressed in a soft voice? Does he or she imitate words more reliably when the adult speaks very slowly?

The therapist can hum, chant or gently sing to communicate to the child, all the while striving to elicit islets of normalcy, such as improved eye contact, less tension in the child's face, more babbling or even word repetition. The practitioner or parent will want to experiment with a range of vocal pitches, tones and rhythms and to pay close attention as to which draw the child closer and which induce the child to pull back from a sense of connection.

The Tactile Channel

Touch is a powerful conduit of relationship and connection. Yet children thought to be autistic typically seek to avoid physical connection with others. How can the practitioner or parent build closeness and initial relationship using the very channel that children with autistiform features so often resist? As Greenspan and Wieder emphasized, one begins by paying close attention to the child's level of sensory sensitivity and reactivity: hypo-, hyper-, or mixed. Their clinical literature is full of creative examples of how the tactile sense can be used to open and close circles of communication.[3] And from the Feuerstein perspective, the tactile channel has the potential to yield islets of normalcy that are related to touch. During initial interactive assessment sessions, the islets yielded through this channel, as through other sensory channels, help inform intervention strategies for creating a playful and warmly interactive treatment approach. Relevant questions include:

- What is the child's response to closeness and touch by an adult? Further avoidance? Or a sense of pleasure and movement toward the adult?
- If touch induces closeness, can the child sustain this closeness for a long time or only fleetingly? Under what circumstances?
- Does the child prefer light gentle touch or deep pressure? What is the effect of varied pressures on the child's vocalizing, eye contact and emotional responsiveness?
- Can gentle tickling be used to release tension or aid eye contact and emotional contact with the child? Or does the child prefer strong tickling?
- Which type of massage induces a sense of greater openness from the child—gentle or firm? To which parts of the body does the child show less resistance to touch?
- Does the child better tolerate gentle or firm holding in the adult's lap?
- What are the child's responses to objects and materials of varying

textures? Are materials with rough, smooth or silky textures more effective in eliciting contact or shared attention?

- How do fluid or squishy materials, like water, sand, mud, play-doh or clay, affect the child's degree of relatedness? What changes in the child's level of responsiveness do such materials catalyze?
- What are the intersensory effects of various materials and textures on the child's degree of responsiveness? Which tactile variations lead to more responsive eye contact? More babbling? More imitative behavior? A sense of emotional closeness?

The Kinesthetic Channel: Movement

Encouraged by DIR strategies, I have found the kinesthetic channel, the movement of the body in space, to be a remarkably vibrant channel for eliciting islets of normalcy, for catalyzing circles of communication and for literally jump-starting a sense of relational closeness. Parents and practitioners will want to note:

- In general, what is the child's degree and style of movement? Slow? Speedy? Fluid? Stiff? Comfortable in his or her body?
- What activities enliven the slow-moving child and propel her into the world? What types of activities calm the hyper child and help him center and inch toward relatedness?
- How does the child respond to gentle versus energetic rocking?
- Can the child be wooed into a game of jumping, which has the potential to trigger a powerful developmental boost?
- Will the child accept being spun around, either when held by the adult or when spun in a vestibular dish? To what degree does the child tolerate or enjoy this? How do kinesthetic activities affect the child's communicative propensity?
- What islets of normalcy are observed if the child is lifted? Engaged in roughhousing?
- What are some of the intersensory effects related to movement and relation of the body in space? For example, do loud noises propel the child into hyperactivity, and thus interfere with the sense of reciprocity with the child?
- How do changes in the child's position (above or below the adult's line of vision) and type of activity affect the child's receptivity? Does eye contact improve if the child is placed above the adult's eye level, for example, by standing the child on the table? Does eye contact improve if the child is active?
- How do changes in placement and type of movement affect the child's vocal, verbal and/or relational output? Does she babble, speak, gesture or point more when active? Is there a difference if the activity arises spontaneously from the child or is induced by the adult?

Dynamic, playfully interactive assessment and treatment sessions require energy on the part of the adult! As the parent or practitioner actively engages the child, questions abound, and the adult maintains a keen eye for answers about the impact of movement, in addition to other sensory channels, on the child's degree and quality of relatedness.

When assessing or treating a child with suspected autism, one of my favorite physical activities involved not only kinesthetic factors but also incorporated vestibular (balance), tactile, visual and auditory channels, the combination of which yielded many opportunities for connectedness. Verbally, via gestures or using light touch I wooed the child into a jumping game in which I stood behind the child, and gently held him or her under the arms. As we both faced the mirror in order to encourage eye contact, I lifted the child gently in a mini-jump. Some children resisted at first, but I gently persisted in lifting them slightly. Most children warmed to this game and as they did I increased the height of the lift and, when appropriate, the strength of the thud with which I returned them to the floor, counting aloud with each jump, up to ten. The hyposensitive children generally needed or preferred a heavier landing. Often initially remote and cut-off children responded with lovely warm eye contact, excited sounds or even words as the jumping game continued. Parents could also be enlisted to gently lift the child, while from the side I coached and pointed out the exciting new islets of normalcy that were emerging from the action. Some children thought to be autistic found this multisensory experience so unexpectedly energizing that they began to vocalize or even to join in the counting.

Another favored activity was to stand the avoidant, nonspeaking child on top of my cleared desktop—always holding on carefully so that the child did not fall. Standing on the floor, I faced the child and dipped slightly with each number as I counted "1, 2, 3, Go!" The dipping helped me to note whether the child was following my slight descent with some eye contact. The "Go!" was said softly or loudly, depending on the child's auditory sensitivity. The child's supported jump onto the carpet could be gentle or hard, depending on the child's perceived preference for a gentle landing or a hard thud. In repeating this activity, it was possible to note whether the child was showing signs of anticipation, an important islet of normalcy, just before liftoff. With children who visibly warmed to the activity, found pleasure in it and delighted in the supported jump, an added gentle tickle before liftoff or an added little twirl before setting the child on the floor offered more opportunities to encourage and gauge responsiveness. The activity repeated as long as the child was involved, engaged and responding. These types of activities, along with the use of a vestibular dish for spinning the child, or a large foam rubber U-shape for rocking the child (such as Annie enjoyed, Chapter 3), proved invaluable in assessing and treating cut-off, nonverbal children. The use of kinesthetic activity so often broke the ice of a child's silence or remoteness, generating many circles of communication, and providing opportunities to identify many islets of normalcy that had not been visible when the child had been stationary or passive.

Play as Pivotal

While islets of normalcy can be sought in any context (dressing, bathing, learning, even during snack time), with young children the predominant context in the search for islets of normalcy is clearly the world of play. Play is a powerful clinical tool. As mentioned in the Introduction, play possesses the developmental power to reach into the interstices of the child's innermost world and abilities. Play involves every aspect of a child's being and it touches every facet of child development: emotion, personality, imagination, attention, speech, thought, social skills and fine and gross motor skills. Through play, children tell us who they are, what they understand, what they feel and what they can and cannot do.

Play functions as a dynamic two-way street for anyone seeking to assist children considered autistic. From an observational stance, a child's play serves as a virtual mirror, reflecting the child's inner world and abilities. The practitioner's "close reading" of the play of a child with autistic symptoms has the potential to reveal the dynamics of where and how the child is blocked, and can also yield exciting glimpses of the child behind the symptoms. From an active, operational stance, play offers the adult interesting and varied opportunities for energetically entering the detached child's world and for catalyzing increasingly sustained connection and communication. Even when the child is not yet playing in any noticeably meaningful way, an adult's sensitively enticing that child toward play interaction on a simple sensory or "baby playtime" level can catalyze a positive developmental turning point. Somewhat like a safari adventurer entering into darkened jungles, the adult observes and/or attempts to enter the reality of the child through the world of play, equipped only with the types of qualitative questions detailed above. The child's responses in increasingly reciprocal activity and communication provide the qualitative answers.

As the reader has surely noticed, a dynamic, playfully interactive assessment or treatment session is not one of quietly observing and seeking symptoms. Rather, the assessor is actively involved in engaging the child playfully in any and all sensory channels with the aim of opening and closing circles of communication as well as observing, eliciting and strengthening islets of normalcy. In the ensuing brief discussion, the focus shifts from the kinds of questions that generate insights related to particular sensory channels to a series of questions related to the general realm of play itself. As in the above sections, many of these questions have been adopted from Floortime guidelines[4]:

- Is the child's approach to play materials purposeful (as in hugging a doll) or stereotypical (as in flapping a doll)? If the child's approach to play materials is stereotypical, can purposeful use be elicited? If so, how?
- Which play materials or activities create a sense of emotional contact with the child? Eye contact? Physical contact? Vocal contact? Verbal contact?

- Which play materials/activities elicit pleasure in contact?
- Which play materials encourage shared attention?
- Can the child be engaged in turn-taking?
- Is there any evidence of symbolic play?
- What play activities encourage babbling, vocalization or speech?
- What play activities help bypass or reduce perseverative behaviors and induce calm and contact?
- Do boisterous play activities, such as jumping or spinning, entice an avoidant child into contact and shared pleasure?
- Can the child solve problems that arise in play, whether concrete problems such as finding a lost ball or symbolic problems such as helping the good guys overcome the bad guys?

At this point, the reader may be wondering: where does the search for islets of normalcy begin with a child who is not yet playing at all? How does one initiate play with a child who cannot yet make interpersonal contact, let alone engage in interactive play? Greenspan and Wieder counseled parents and practitioners to begin at the beginning, developmentally speaking. That is, to use sensorily attuned activities such as intriguing infant toys, a game of peek-a-boo, tickling, blowing bubbles for the child to pop—all of these in order to begin to woo the avoidant child into contact.

A meaningful, descriptive play-based dynamic assessment of a child with autistiform symptoms may begin with an activity as simple as blowing bubbles, jumping with the child, releasing a rubber-band propelled "helicopter" to entice the interest of the child or, as in the case of a child who presents at a higher stage of development, providing the props for symbolic play. Play activities may range from active, sensory-motor play—such as tickling, swinging, rocking, cuddling, jumping—to quietly drawing the child into connection using interesting cause-and-effect toys such as a ball that lights up or a musical jack-in-the-box.

Important information can be gleaned, first by careful observation and then by actively using play to elicit and expand contact. Via play activity, a clinician may notice that a child's lack of eye contact may not be absolute. The quality of eye contact may change from avoidant or seemingly indifferent to a look of curiosity and delight when bubbles are introduced. Through the "safety" of a screen of bubbles, the child might even be prepared to risk a little direct eye contact with the practitioner. Similarly, a silent child may suddenly burst into excited babbling when lifted repeatedly in front of a mirror, enjoying the brief sense of weightless freedom. The excitement of being lifted can even surprise a child out of an avoidant repertoire into warmly shared laughter. Sammy's jumping off my desk (Chapter 10) is an example of how action triggered language. Also, children thought to be autistic may reveal that they possess an incipient sense of self and an understanding of an empathic relationship when they show an interest in symbolic play (for example, in an activity as simple as their offering a bottle to the doll).

It is primarily through play, in my experience, that examples of non-symptomatic or even normative behavior can be found, and a sense of connection, whether nonverbal, vocal or verbal, can be made with the child. It is play that enables us to move beyond misleading assumptions and statistical summation to achieve dynamic contact with the child. Play materials and activities offer virtually limitless opportunities for making contact, entering the child's inner affective world, and exploring the potential modifiability of autistiform symptoms. Painstaking observation of the child coupled with active play can provide a much clearer picture of a child's developmental strengths, weaknesses, avenues for emotional connection and evidence for the modifiability of symptoms than instruments which sum symptoms as uniform, unchangeable entities. By applying the type of play-based assessment summarized here, it has been possible to look beyond the presenting diagnoses and to discern clearer explanations, causes and treatment options for the children's presentations.

The silent reflections of the clinician during the observation phase of play-based dynamic/qualitative assessment might be something like: "This child has been in the room for twenty minutes and has not yet looked at me, but he looked at his parents briefly. When Dad took out a musical toy, the child smiled in recognition. The child is purposeful as he digs through Mom's purse for a candy. Mom's humming relaxes the child and evokes a little more eye contact." One observes carefully how and when islets of normalcy appear, no matter how faintly, and under what conditions symptoms diminish in intensity or frequency. The answers to these questions are not meant to be summed and scored. The answers are meant to be noted, qualitatively nuanced, processed in detail by the practitioner, and then used to formulate practical recommendations for parents with the aim of strengthening the child behind the symptoms.

The above lists of questions are not exhaustive—many more such nuanced questions will arise in the process of searching for islets of normalcy. Beyond the answers to the above listings of questions lies yet another layer of more general questions:

- What is the approximate ratio of strengths to weaknesses in the child's profile? Do islets of normalcy predominate? Or does the child appear to be drowning in a sea of symptoms, with few islets of normalcy in sight? If so, how can the assessing practitioner generate more islets?
- Across a series of assessment or treatment sessions, how is this ratio changing? Are islets gradually coalescing into "continents"? If so, what is helping this happen? If not, what might be impeding the process?
- What is the intensity of effort needed to detect, elicit and/or sustain islets of normalcy? For example, after a gentle tickle, does language stream from the child? Or is each babble, repeated sound, word or sentence emitted only after intense effort on the part of the adult?
- Across a series of sessions, are the intensity, degree and type of effort needed to elicit islets changing? Is it getting easier to reach the child?

• As the child improves, and as new islets accrue and existing islets strengthen, what new strategies or therapies must be added to meet the child's improved situation and help the child progress further?

Finally, there are other important questions whose answers impact on the complex interplay between the observed islets of normalcy, the child's potential modifiability and the child's actual prognosis and progress: to what degree do the child's parents have the emotional and physical energy, time and resources needed to move the child meaningfully from his or her current presentation?

Our work at the Institute took place in the real world, with parents who were exhausted raising a family that included a child with special needs, who due to work schedules often lacked the time required to apply play strategies or to take children to any additional therapies, and/or who lacked the financial resources to provide those therapies. The playful work of searching for islets of normalcy that took place in my office was often exciting, even exhilarating, when the child showed glimmers, and even more, of responding and relating. Yet our recommendations to the parents had to be sensitively attuned to the parents' realities. Were they able to share the excitement of observing these modest, even miniscule, changes? Or were they still so burdened by worry and doubt about their child's abilities that they could not yet internalize the potential impact of a different way of working with their child? Had I adequately helped them understand the developmental importance of these newly evident islets of normalcy? Did the parents realistically have the energy, time and the financial means needed to translate our recommendations into reality? And if the answer to any of these questions was "no," then supporting the parents toward participating in what was for them a new paradigm became an important focus in the follow-up sessions with the child. If parental energy, time and/or financial resources were limited, then the challenge was to try to help them piece together a "developmental first aid" program that was feasible for their situation, one that contained the optimal services, educational settings, supports and treatments to help their child progress under these less than ideal circumstances.

Case Vignettes

The following case vignettes of Amy, Gordie and Leo illustrate how thinking along the sensory channels in a play milieu, as advocated in Floortime practice, opens worlds of functional understanding and potential communication with difficult-to-reach children. They also illustrate the excitement and promise that identifying islets of normalcy generate. Amy, Gordie and Leo, each in his or her own way, illustrate different applications of utilizing various sensory modalities with challenging children, and how the play focus led to positive results during initial meetings.

Amy and Gordie were each seen once, Leo twice. In each of these cases, I felt privileged to catch glimpses of the child behind the symptoms, followed by a sense of sadness at not having been able to help realize and witness the further emergence of these children, whose progress for varying reasons was not followed further. So these three vignettes reflect the excitement of eliciting those first islets of normalcy as well as the poignancy of an unfinished story.

Amy: Eye Contact and Rhythmic Movement

Five-year-old Amy had been diagnosed as autistic at a child development clinic. She was profoundly deaf. This somewhat forlorn looking little girl entered my office with her mother. Her clothes were unkempt and dirty. Her young mother appeared discouraged, even depressed, at having a child who was profoundly deaf and recently diagnosed with autism as well. I wondered whether the child's physical appearance reflected her mother's degree of discouragement.

I was faced with a particularly difficult challenge: how to find and elicit islets of normalcy, and how to open and close circles of communication, with a child who could not hear. Amy did not know sign language, nor did I for that matter. In dynamic assessment sessions I often used my voice as a means of reaching a nonverbal child—by playfully using a lower or higher tone and pitch of voice, or emitting car crash sounds to spur a child to engage in car play with me, or perhaps singing or humming as I gently rocked or tickled a child, as well as many other vocal strategies. But this entire avenue of entry was blocked—for Amy and for me. I felt extremely limited as to how to engage this child, who did not yet exhibit task orientation abilities. She had been placed among low functioning autistic youngsters where, it could be inferred, the staff's expectations for her and her peers were low. Her functional skills had not been developed to the point that Amy might sit at the table and purposefully construct a puzzle, match pictures, color or even play with dolls. Her demeanor communicated that she had not been worked with effectively.

Amy wandered around my small office but did not engage purposefully with any of the play materials scattered about the room. I noticed that her physical coordination was good. There were no traces of stereotypical flapping, rocking or circuit-walking behavior. Even more encouraging, her eye contact with me was wary but generally open and steady. She did not approach her mother for comfort in this strange situation. A sign of being cut off? I wondered whether Amy's distance from her mother had anything to do with Amy's sensing her mother's feelings of discouragement, helplessness and hopelessness.

I knew what I wanted to do: to open and close circles of communication, in DIR parlance, and to identify and elicit islets of normalcy, as per Feuerstein. But it was not clear how to accomplish this. At one point Amy lay on her back on the carpet. I knelt down near her feet, facing her. Perhaps here was an opportunity. Amy's eye contact remained engaged with mine. Gently I took hold of her feet, and slowly bent her knees, moving them back toward her chest, so that I was leaning toward her face. Amy pushed me back with her feet. I gently leaned in toward her again. Again Amy pushed me back. There was something purposeful and communicative in what she was doing, as if she was signaling with her feet and legs, "I know that we have a little movement dialogue going here."

We continued with this little game for a few minutes as I tried to think how to expand this rudimentary movement dialogue. I decided to use rhythmic patterns—such as, quick, quick, quick, pause. I pushed Amy's bent knees, alternating right and left, in time to this rhythm, repeating the cadence several times: quick, quick, quick, pause; quick, quick, quick, pause. I decided to test whether Amy was literally coming along for the ride as I moved her knees back and forth or whether she had actually internalized the pattern. I initiated: quick, quick ... Amy completed the movement sequence: quick, pause! For a while longer I continued this interaction with her, creating little movement cadences with her legs as I gazed into her eyes, and she gazed steadily back.

Amy had demonstrated that she had discerned rhythmic patterns in what she could have misinterpreted as my arbitrary movements. She was clearly participating in these movement dialogues, closing and opening circles of communication, all the while maintaining meaningful eye contact. Her conscious participation in this soundless game indicated to me that Amy possessed as yet undeveloped intelligence. She needed to be taught sign language. She needed to learn to sit and enjoy a wide variety of cognitive table tasks. She needed to be taught to read. None of this had happened to date.

I ruled out autism. Amy was too present, too in touch and too communicative in her eye contact and in her conscious participation in our movement dialogue. She was not a cut-off personality—only a child suffering extreme isolation and underdevelopment due to her profound deafness. During my many years at the Institute, I encountered many children who had been misdiagnosed as autistic spectrum and whose backgrounds included mild to moderate hearing loss, often due to ear infections and fluids. Amy's hearing loss was the most profound I encountered. Her lack of language, her lack of social skills and her undeveloped task orientation had been misinterpreted as autism. Seeking islets of normalcy and creating circles of communication using the visual and movement channels had opened the door to worlds of intelligence and abilities yet to be developed in Amy.

I explained to her mother my reasoning for concluding that Amy was not autistic. I attempted to help her understand the significance of Amy's conscious participation in our communicative movement game—that her participation indicated awareness and a healthy intelligence yet to be developed. Explaining to Amy's mother that the mandate of the Institute was to provide further assessment sessions and to follow and support Amy's progress, I suggested that we arrange another meeting. We did so, but Amy never returned to the Institute. Sadly, I concluded that the tiny glimmer of hope in Amy's potential which I tried to convey was not enough to encourage her mother, who was so burdened by feelings of deep discouragement. There were days when I felt inadequate to the task. To have glimpsed evidence of Amy's potential but not to have been able to accompany her on the journey to realization of her potential was disappointing. That the mother's discouragement stemmed from a misdiagnosis of autism made my disappointment even keener.

Gordie: Eye Contact, Movement and Gentle Touch

Years ago I was invited abroad to lecture on the combination of Feuerstein's educational philosophy and playful DIR strategies that had proven effective in assessing and treating children with suspected autism. On the third day of the visit, after two days of lecturing, I was meant to work individually with several children considered autistic, while their parents and a few therapists observed from behind the large mirrored glass. To add to the immense pressure, since arriving I had contracted laryngitis, and had whispered my three-hour presentation into a hastily arranged microphone. On that third day I had absolutely no voice, and the children and their parents were waiting.

Gordie was the last child that day. His mother and a few of his therapists were observing us from behind the observation mirror. A lovely four-year-old who had been diagnosed as autistic, Gordie did not speak during our session. His eye contact was poor at the outset, but his body language did not communicate excess tension, nor did he exhibit any stereotypical flapping or rocking behaviors. Gordie seemed comfortable in his body. Despite his quietness and his iffy eye contact, Gordie seemed very present.

Gordie found himself a comfortable niche in the soft beanbag chair and settled in, not communicating either verbally or nonverbally any need for connection, interaction or purposeful activity. Gordie did not appear stubborn—he was just sitting there, watching me, but effectively avoiding direct eye contact if I glanced his way. Yet he possessed a strong and positive presence, and I sensed within a lovely little boy. But the question was how to reach him, given his low energy and my missing voice?

I made several active attempts to engage Gordie in play, and as I did so, I whispered to him, "This puzzle makes music! . . . Here comes the car . . . vroom . . . Now I'm going to look for more toys for you." After clearly failing to interest Gordie in various play materials, I calmed, centered and thought developmental thoughts: "He's in there. He just needs to be met right where he is. Go back to something more primal. Use touch for starters."

I knelt down in front of the beanbag chair where Gordie was ensconced. He was not yet looking at me. I told Gordie in a barely audible whisper that I was going to take off his shoes. I kept my gaze toward him steady and soft, with a gentle smile on my face. If he happened to look my way, perhaps this would help reduce any sense of threat. As I slowly removed his shoes, Gordie began to look at me. I ever so gently rubbed the soles of his stockinged feet. Intrigued, and hopefully enjoying the light touch, Gordie watched me as I stroked each foot in turn.

He was with me. With his gaze Gordie was closing a circle of communication that began with my touch. At the same time, his now steady gaze opened a circle of communication, impelling me to continue and to chain these many circles to lengthen the duration of this fragile visual and emotional engagement.

I slowly began to lean from side to side as I stroked the soles of his feet. Gordie maintained eye contact. His glance even shifted, watching me as I slowly leaned to the left, then right. I continued to whisper to Gordie: "Oh. That feels so nice. Now your left foot. Now your right foot." I wondered whether it was possible to expand and deepen the incipient sense of connection with Gordie.

I whispered to Gordie that now I was going to take off his socks. Ever so slowly, so that Gordie would not retreat, I removed his socks and continued the sideways rocking movement, holding and stroking each foot in turn as he now gazed at me steadily. Although terribly self-conscious that there were many eyes watching from the other side of the glass, and wondering how clean Gordie's feet were, I decided to continue rocking from side to side, but at the end of each leaning arc to say "kiss!" and to kiss gently the sole of each foot in turn.

I tried to keep my voice, rocking movements, intensity and even the timing of each kiss controlled and gentle, with no sudden spurts of energy that might frighten him and cause him to look away. There was an almost hypnotic quality about the intensity of this quiet, intimate interaction with Gordie, both for him and for me. Gordie gazed steadfastly, following the alternating direction of each kissed foot. This rocking and kissing activity continued for perhaps seven to ten minutes. By then, it was time to end the session.

There had been a small but significant breakthrough. Gordie's initial apparent indifference to contact, tinged perhaps with some resignation or possibly even depression, had been penetrated. He was there, needy and waiting. I told Gordie that I had enjoyed playing with him but soon we would be finishing and that his mother would be coming in to help him put his shoes on and to take him home.

What ensued was both dramatic and moving. Having already reviewed the developmental information his parents had submitted, I had met with Gordie's mother briefly before the session with him. She had appeared to be the very picture of sadness, overwhelmed by the feeling that she had lost her child to autism.

Now she entered the room to put on Gordie's shoes. Something within her had changed! She appeared almost moved to tears. There was a sense of determination about her, missing earlier in the day. She knelt down where Gordie still lay in the beanbag chair and talked to him directly, "Come on, Gordie. Let's get those shoes and socks on. Give me your foot. Great. Now give me the other. Now I'll help you with your coat and we'll go home to Daddy."

When Gordie had received the diagnosis of autism, this mother evidently had lost much hope for him and his future. She had also lost confidence in her own abilities to connect with her son. Overcome by a sense of resignation, she had essentially negated her own sense of the abilities and personality of the little boy she loved—and likely had warmly interacted with—as she saw his future carried along the river of what appeared to her to be a dark diagnosis. She had devalued her own intuitive way of relating to her child, doubted her own ability to relate to and care for her own child, and submitted all her hopes and expectations to the power of an autism diagnosis.

Such profound self-doubt in a parent's own feelings, abilities and even affection for their child with autistiform symptoms, sadly, is not uncommon. Most commonly, I have observed that the parent's emotional plunge occurs precisely at the time when the young child is most in need of mother's energy and love. Seeking islets of normalcy and creating circles of communication are necessary not only to assess and treat the child, but also to provide parents with initial evidence of their child's ability to change. With such evidence before them, many parents begin to feel more hopeful and encouraged.

The energy, conviction and warmth with which Gordie's mother talked to him as she put on his shoes conveyed that something, unexpectedly, had shifted within her. Observing from the other side of the glass, she had evidently realized that her Gordie was still in there, he could be talked to, he could be reached and that she had much to give him as a mother.

The play work with Gordie demonstrates how the visual, movement and tactile channels were used in tandem to open and close circles of communication, and to elicit islets of normalcy. Gordie would need continued intensive DIR intervention. From this single session, it was clear that his situation was far from hopeless. I left the country a few days later and was not able to follow his progress in any way. I can only hope that Gordie received the recommended interactive play strategies of DIR and that he is now a competent young adult.

Leo: Overcoming a Visual and Auditory Addiction

Leo's first session at the Institute was a supreme challenge that confronted me with a steep learning curve. Aged five-and-a-half and bearing a diagnosis of autism, Leo was in profound developmental trouble, evident in many realms. He did not make eye contact with me, and rarely with his parents. He did not speak. He made some vocal and sub-vocal humming sounds, but that was all. His body was very stiff and he sometimes rocked a bit from side to side. Often he held his arms up in a "w" position, sometimes flapping them. He appeared frail and delicate, short and slight for his chronological age. I noticed that his fingers were extremely slender, and that his hands and fingers were smaller than expected in a five-year-old. I made a mental note to suggest to his parents a genetic workup.

As noted in other chapters, Professor Feuerstein considered genes to be influences but not the ultimate determinants of human potential. The detection of a genetic aberration need not necessarily seal a child's fate. On the positive side of the ledger, the identification of a genetic influence sometimes helps lift parents from any sense of self-blame or inadequacy that they might have taken on in response to the child's difficulties and the challenges of raising him.

By far the most problematic aspect of Leo's presentation was his intensely obsessive interest in his parents' cellphones. Leo was completely fixated, hypnotized by the screen of the cellphone he held while rocking to the rhythm of the music. He was cut off and far away from interpersonal interaction. It was clear why he had come to be diagnosed as autistic. In fact, he was one of the few children that I saw during twenty-five years at the Institute whom I would consider genuinely autistic.

His parents reported that whenever Leo was denied access to a cellphone, he screamed with rage. Interestingly, however, Leo did not scream or rage when at his special kindergarten for autistic children, even though in that setting he lacked access to a cellphone.

The therapists in his kindergarten were frustrated by Leo's lack of progress and had recommended that Leo be placed in a setting among more seriously impaired children. Leo's parents were not convinced that his special education setting for autistic children was to his benefit, but they were baffled and frustrated by his difficulties and uncertain as to what his educational needs were. Aware that the Feuerstein Institute worked from an unconventional psychological and developmental outlook, they were hopeful that we could shed some light on Leo's situation.

During my first session with Leo, I made no progress penetrating Leo's fixated isolation. I tried unsuccessfully to lure him away from the cellphone screen by using bubbles, balloons, musical toys—all without success. Sensing that the only way to reach the Leo behind the symptoms was to deprive him of the visual obsession of the cellphone, and thus possibly startle him into contact with the real world, I raised the issue with his parents. They were all too familiar with the prolonged screaming protest that would be unleashed. At home they usually obliged Leo by letting him play with their cellphones, in the interest of a quieter home life.

Before attempting to dislodge Leo from the phone, or vice versa, I would have to explain to his parents that the inevitable distress that Leo would exhibit would not harm him but might ultimately help him, leaving his visual and auditory senses freer and more available to the world. I explained to them that on his next visit to the Institute, I would like to see Leo without access to a cellphone. I told them that I anticipated that Leo's reaction would be one of great distress, but that the expression of this distress—with his protest itself an islet of normalcy—could help Leo open up to the world. His parents were open to trying this "cellphonectomy" during their next visit to the Institute.

On his second visit, Leo's father waited outside the office with the cellphone while Leo's mother accompanied him inside. His mother remained with him in the office. With her full consent, I locked my office door in order to passively contain the emotional havoc I anticipated.

Deprived of the distraction or perhaps defense of a cellphone and in a state of heightened anxiety in a still strange situation, Leo did not disappoint. He raged, screamed and cried for a long time. Through it, I tried to give his mother some emotional support—that Leo was not in danger, that there was no harm to him in his distress, and that his separation from the phone had the potential to release Leo from a visual and auditory obsession, a kind of addiction in fact, that was crippling his development. My proposed strategy was marginally in tune with some Floortime strategies in which therapists are often encouraged to gently counter a silent child's wishes or to play dumb in order to elicit active resistance and anger—which in itself is a communicative response. As a child psychologist, I was comfortable entering the depths of this child's distress and understood how to support him through it.

Relying on my experience in play therapy as Leo raged, I remained genuinely empathic. In gentle tones, I verbally reflected to him: "Yes, you are so upset and sad. I know you are angry about not having the cellphone to hold. It's good to cry when we are sad." His rage, fear and anxiety began to subside. Gradually, there appeared shorter, then longer, breaks in his tantrum. He appeared to be listening to my voice now and then. There were definite instances of eye contact, almost "aha" experiences for him as he fleetingly recognized that there was a world out there, and that perhaps it was not as terrible as he might fear.

Leo's trance-like, obsessive, perseverative behavior had been part of him for a long time. It was not possible in a single session to transform his overall profile from totally closed to somewhat open. However, this intense interaction with him did demonstrate that it was possible to observe that his being separated from the cellphone (under supported circumstances) was a positive direction, if there was to be any hope for his development. His mother had observed the proceedings, and she understood their significance. I recommended that the parents steel their courage and begin a process of gradual reduction of phone time, while at the same time be ready to empathically and warmly communicate with him verbally, without panicking at his degree of anger.

I took the recommendations further. For years my practical experience in educational settings while an undergraduate in Boston and later a doctoral intern in Vancouver, BC, had exposed me to the developmental benefits of educational integration (inclusion) for special needs children. Properly carried out with supportive, trained staff, integration aides when needed, and additional therapies either on site or after school, I had seen that educational inclusion was often the crucial factor in strengthening a special needs child. Immersed in what Feuerstein termed a "modifying environment,"[5,6] the special needs child is thus exposed to normative models of language, communication, play, learning and socialization by typical peers whose energy has the potential to pull the special needs child forward. As per the recommendations of his current special kindergarten staff, Leo was headed for precisely the opposite—an educational demotion, a transfer to a setting in which he would be surrounded by even lower functioning children, with the risk that the performance expectations of the staff might be lower as well.

At the end of this second session, Leo's parents listened to my rationale for recommending educational inclusion in a typical setting with an integration aide—an admittedly unconventional move given his unique presentation. They understood that he would require additional therapies, including intensive DIR intervention, outside kindergarten hours. To my surprise his parents were open to this recommendation. Given the current prevalence in the Israeli school system of special classes for special needs children, his parents and I knew that they faced an uphill struggle to find such an inclusive placement for Leo and to receive the approval for this from the educational authorities.

In my report to the parents, I recommended educational integration, with an aide for Leo, in a regular kindergarten among children one to two years younger than him. In that report, I acknowledged that on the surface such a direction might appear counterintuitive, given Leo's intensely idiosyncratic presentation. At the same time, I outlined the enormous potential advantage for his development: the plentiful opportunities to be drawn forward by the current of healthy developmental energy of typical children, who would then serve as healthy role models for speech and shared activity. For Leo, without spoken language, lacking motivation and tools for social contact, and unable to play meaningfully, immersion among typical children would be a shock to his system at first. But, if he were supported by an integration aide, that immersion within a normative environment might just help move him toward life.

His parents and I knew that these recommendations would be considered farfetched and even inappropriate in some circles: "Doesn't this psychologist see how seriously impaired this child is?" Indeed, I had seen how seriously impaired Leo was. His auditory and visual channels for contact had been completely blocked by his obsessive fixation with the cellphone screen. However, by depriving Leo of the phone for a short time, I had seen that those channels could be opened. Leo had raged, but he had also cried, expressing emotion. He had made some eye contact as he looked at the source of his rage—me. His cries and vocalizations of protest at being deprived had been highly expressive. With this expressive rage, he was no longer cut off. He was communicating.

Leo's parents and I were not overly optimistic that a welcoming typical kindergarten setting could be found for him, given the proclivity of the educational system in Israel for special classes for children with special needs. They understood that this bold recommendation might not ultimately be realized. Yet they were prepared to try to find such a setting for him. At the very least, his parents and I hoped that my recommendation for his educational inclusion would serve as a strong counterweight to the proposal from his current special class teacher to demote Leo to a placement among lower functioning children. In a follow-up phone call, Leo's mother informed me that she was seriously looking for a regular kindergarten that might be willing to accept Leo with an aide.

As mentioned above, Leo's parents never returned to the Institute. Despite the frustration of not knowing how this child's story unfolded, I opted to include Leo in this casebook because he serves as an important example of how islets of normalcy can be elicited and identified along sensory channels within the profiles of even seriously cut off and, on the face of it, very impaired autistic children. Some might argue that a genuinely autistic child like Leo is by definition unchangeable. Yet even the strong autistic shell of this child began to crack. How I would have loved to coax the little sparks of emotion and contact that began to emerge into a warm flame of developmental energy.

Notes

1 Anna Jean Ayers, "Characteristics of Types of Sensory Integrative Dysfunction," *American Journal of Occupational Therapy* 25 (1971): 329–34.
2 Stanley I. Greenspan and Serena Wieder, *The Child with Special Needs* (Reading, MA: Addison-Wesley, 1998).
3 Ibid.
4 Ibid.
5 Reuven Feuerstein, "Shaping Modifying Environments through Inclusion," *Transylvanian Journal of Psychology*, Special Issue No. 2 (2007): 9–23.
6 Reuven Feuerstein and Yaakov Rand, *You Love Me!! Don't Accept Me as I Am: Helping the Low-Functioning Person Excel* (Jerusalem: ICELP, 2006).

References

Ayers, Anna Jean. "Characteristics of Types of Sensory Integrative Dysfunction." *American Journal of Occupational Therapy* 25 (1971): 329–34.
Feuerstein, Reuven. "Shaping Modifying Environments through Inclusion." *Transylvanian Journal of Psychology*, Special Issue No. 2 (2007): 9–23.
Feuerstein, Reuven and Yaakov Rand. *You Love Me!! Don't Accept Me as I Am: Helping the Low-Functioning Person Excel*. Jerusalem: ICELP, 2006.
Greenspan, Stanley I. and Serena Wieder. *The Child with Special Needs*. Reading, MA: Addison-Wesley, 1998.

13 The *DSM* on Autism

A Closer Look

Nearly all the children presenting with autistiform symptoms whom I assessed in dynamic, play-based interactive fashion at the Feuerstein Institute had been previously assessed and diagnosed elsewhere as PDD, AD or ASD at clinics and hospitals in Israel and abroad. In those clinics the staff specializing in autism had invariably used as the accepted gold standard of diagnosis the autism criteria of the now obsolete *DSM-IV-TR*[1] or the current *DSM-5*.[2] Aware that the Feuerstein methods of assessment, intervention and understanding of the process of developmental change, with an emphasis on potential, were qualitatively different from those of a conventional psychological perspective, most of the parents sought a second opinion from the Institute regarding the accuracy of their child's autism-related diagnosis, insights regarding their child's prognosis and additional recommendations and strategies to help their child.

The former *DSM-IV-TR* and the current *DSM-5* criteria for autism are broadly and flexibly configured. I have observed that these generously configured criteria present a considerable risk of yielding what is known in research circles as false positives; that is, for example, the equivalent of test results showing that a woman is pregnant when she is not. I routinely shared with parents the formal *DSM* autism criteria to help them understand how easy it is for a conscientious practitioner to arrive at a falsely positive diagnosis of autism—formerly AD or PDD-NOS and currently ASD—even when that practitioner has applied the criteria scrupulously. Engaging parents in a brief close reading of the formal autism diagnostic criteria helped create a readiness and an openness to begin working dynamically with their child's difficulties and, above all, latent abilities. This close reading also helped parents realize that the diagnosis their child had received need not necessarily be a determinant of who their child is and what their child may yet become.

Since the first *DSM* was published in 1952,[3] every fifteen years or so the criteria for the numerous diagnoses it details undergo a thorough revision, with occasional interim revisions. The criteria for the diagnosis of autism have not remained static over time. Over the years I found it productive to share with parents not only the details but also the implications of the formal criteria which had been used elsewhere to diagnose their child. We did more than read the criteria together. We probed them, and together we pondered some of the challenges these formal criteria contain. What follows is a close reading of the autism criteria of the former *DSM-IV-TR* and the current *DSM-5*, the two editions relevant to the children whose stories are told in this book. For this close reading, we will use a conceptual magnifying glass to put these criteria, their details and their implications under a higher resolution. Although the *DSM-IV-TR* is no longer in use, I have included the close reading of its autism criteria in order to provide a contextual backdrop for the current *DSM-5* autism criteria. The aim here is to elucidate the phraseology that has sometimes clouded rather than clarified practitioners' and parents' conclusions about children who appear to be autistic. The criteria for AD and ASD are presented here in *paraphrased* form. The *verbatim* criteria for autism from the *DSM-IV-TR* and the current *DSM-5* are reprinted with permission in Appendices I and II, respectively.

The *DSM-IV-TR* and Autism

During the era of the *DSM-IV-TR*, an autism diagnosis was determined by attention to three clusters of possible impairments: qualitative impairments in social interaction, qualitative impairments in communication, and perseverative behaviors. Each cluster was comprised of four possible symptom types.

The cluster which related to qualitative impairments in social interaction included the symptom types:

- Impairments in using nonverbal behaviors such as eye contact or gestures.
- A failure to develop age-appropriate peer relationships.
- A lack of spontaneously seeking to share enjoyment and interests with others.
- A lack of social/emotional reciprocity.

The cluster related to qualitative impairments in communication included:

- Delay in, or lack of, the development of spoken language (assuming the child did not use other modes of communication).
- Serious impairment in initiating or sustaining a conversation.
- Stereotyped, repetitive and/or idiosyncratic language.
- A lack of spontaneous make-believe or social imitative play.

The cluster that addressed restricted repetitive and stereotyped patterns of behavior, interests and activities included:

- Stereotypical behaviors appearing with abnormal intensity or focus.
- Rigid adherence to nonfunctional routines or rituals.
- Stereotyped, repetitive motor mannerisms.
- Preoccupation with parts of objects.

To receive a diagnosis of Autistic Disorder using these former *DSM-IV-TR* criteria the child required six of the twelve possible symptoms in the following array: at least two symptoms related to qualitative impairments in social interaction, at least one symptom related to qualitative impairments in communication and at least one symptom from the category related to restricted repetitive and stereotyped patterns of behavior. These four basic symptoms plus two additional symptoms from any of the three impairment categories then confirmed an autism diagnosis at the time.

Our close reading reveals a number of difficulties with these criteria, which at first glance might appear to have captured the essence of autism. These difficulties, to be elaborated, include a lack of specificity regarding the degree of qualitative impairment required, a functional interrelationship between the communication and social interaction symptom groups and even somewhat with the group of perseverative symptoms, and an emphasis on behavioral manifestations which overlooked any dynamic, clinical, causative roots of the observable behaviors.

The first two groups of symptoms speak of *qualitative* impairments. The critical reader is immediately confronted with a huge problem, so obvious and yet so frequently overlooked as to remind one of the familiar "elephant in the room" image. The degree of qualitative impairment is *not denoted* in any way. Is the practitioner seeking a serious, blatant impairment in social functioning? Does a mild or minor communication impairment qualify? Something in between? How much "qualitative" is considered "impaired"? The practitioner is not informed. This puts us in a difficult place in terms of analysis, with no tools for discretion other than that the child presents with a social communication problem and/or symptoms of "qualitative communication impairment." The potential expansiveness of "qualitative impairments" appears to be far from the succinct focus on emotional cutoffness, or extreme aloneness, and obsessive insistence on sameness that Kanner identified.[4]

As a psychologist who has worked for years detecting qualitative distinctions in children's presentations, I am more than comfortable with qualitative descriptions. Rich descriptions can illumine our clinical understanding, and qualitative distinctions in symptom presentations can serve as an effective basis for designing interventions to enhance a child's strengths. "Qualitative impairments," which may range from the lightest to the most severe, can be described in detail, analyzed and appreciated as a basis for understanding the child's functional presentation and for planning individually-tailored effective interventions. However, the notion of "qualitative impairments" presents challenges when attempting to ascertain a diagnosis based on summing symptoms. That is, discerning and *describing* a child's qualitative impairments is enormously helpful clinically, but *tallying* six out of twelve qualitative impairments as a way of confirming an autism diagnosis is problematic.

Another difficulty that emerges is that the impairments in social interaction and those of communication, and to a degree those of stereotypical behavior, are functionally linked. They are interrelated, interactive, always mutually impacting on one another. Why is that a problem? Because a child with any of a wide range of social communication problems—for example, a child who cannot initiate or maintain a conversation, or who presents with a language delay—will necessarily then encounter problems in social interaction, thus skewing the point score that was needed in the *DSM-IV-TR* to confirm an autistic condition.

Yet there are many reasons that a child may have difficulty initiating a conversation. For example, an emotional problem could easily lead to a situation whereby a child plays alone and appears to be perseverative. Consider also a traumatized child, who may be emotionally imploded and largely silent, limiting her eye contact, refraining from verbal interaction and avoiding social interaction with her kindergarten peers. It may be more comforting for her to stay in the doll corner, continually rocking a baby doll. Similarly, social problems often arise for a child with severe oral dyspraxia who will naturally have difficulty in the actual production of words (as Max, Chapter 7). Seeing his peers cheerfully interact verbally, and comprehending that he, for reasons unknown to him, simply cannot move his mouth and lips to create the words he understands, the child could quite logically decide to play largely on his own and to avoid peers. So he remains in the block corner, constructing circuits for his racing cars to travel along repeatedly. Applying the *DSM-IV-TR* criteria, each of these children could potentially have qualified for an Autistic Disorder diagnosis—yet incorrectly so.

There is a related difficulty in the fact that all of the autism criteria relied on strict behavioral manifestations: the child does or does not initiate, speak, play, flap hands and so on. While on the face of it, this seems a safe and correct way of assessing—looking at clear-cut behaviors—there is an embedded problem with the focus solely on behavior. As will be elaborated later, there is no attention to causation, to the many plausible roots below the surface of the behavioral expressions of a child's difficulties. An abused child, shy and hesitant to speak, who does not approach peers and who prefers to build block towers in kindergarten could easily, mistakenly, have garnered six of the twelve points needed at the time for an autism diagnosis; similarly, a child with undetected or underappreciated hearing problems (such as Davie, Chapter 4).

Other possibilities for an overly liberal use of these former autism criteria abound. A child with a communication problem, for whatever reasons, may prefer his or her own company and the solace of repetitive play over the risk-taking that the world of friendship demands. A highly intelligent gifted child, who at the age of four loves reading about astronomy, may find little in common with his peers and may talk incessantly about Jupiter. Are these children necessarily autistic or "spectrum"? Not necessarily at all. Are such children at risk for being *diagnosed* as autistic? Given the expansive usage, and the elasticity of the former and current official diagnostic autism criteria, very much so, as the stories of Jack, Annie, Davie, Max, Josh and others illustrate.

The criteria for several other disorders that fell under the category of Pervasive Developmental Disorder were then detailed: Rett's Disorder,

Childhood Disintegrative Disorder, and Asperger's Disorder. The final section of the *category* of Pervasive Developmental Disorder presented the *diagnostic* criteria for Pervasive Developmental Disorder Not Otherwise Specified, including Atypical Autism. Known in the field as PDD-NOS, this diagnostic alternative reigned for years. The now obsolete *DSM-IV-TR* description of Pervasive Developmental Disorder Not Otherwise Specified including Atypical Autism 299.80 follows verbatim:

> This category should be used when there is a severe and pervasive impairment in the development of reciprocal social interaction or verbal and nonverbal communication skills, or when stereotyped behavior, interests, and activities are present, but the criteria are not met for a specific Pervasive Developmental Disorder, Schizophrenia, Schizotypal Personality Disorder, or Avoidant Personality Disorder. For example, this category includes "atypical autism"—presentations that do not meet the criteria for Autistic Disorder because of late age of onset, atypical symptomatology, or subthreshold symptomatology or all of these.

> *Reprinted with permission from the Diagnostic and Statistical Manual of Mental Disorders, Fourth Edition Text Revision, (Copyright © 2000). American Psychiatric Association. All Rights Reserved.*

Lecturing to parents and practitioners during the heyday of this diagnosis, I often discussed this diagnostic option with my listeners, asking for their understanding of its meaning and intent. Typically, listeners said that they found the paragraph confusing, ambiguous and unclear. I, too, had to admit that I could not decipher the clinical distinctions. The statement that this category "includes atypical autism" was perplexing. If, as I have suggested, the criteria in the *DSM-IV-TR* for "typical" Autistic Disorder were elastic, interrelated and prone to yielding false positives, what did "atypical" autism mean? The gist seems to be that children who did not fit any of the other above-cited disorders could have been diagnosed as PDD-NOS. Was this then really a diagnosis? It was used as such.

I often asked my listeners to imagine that they were suffering from a nagging cough and had decided to go to the doctor. The doctor then examines them and informs them that they have "Coughing Disorder-NOS." Would they accept such a diagnosis at face value? Any patient would surely want to know whether the condition is a symptom of a cold, bronchitis, pneumonia, an allergic reaction, asthma or a serious disease.

In the field of medicine, physicians have access to refined medical tests to reach a diagnosis. The term PDD-NOS, our close reading reveals, could not offer diagnostic clarity because it was a highly generalized rubric. Since the description of PDD-NOS appeared within a grouping of diagnoses associated with autism, I observed that the term was often used in clinical practice synonymously for developmental conditions which ranged from "mild autism" to classical autism (as per Kanner), and beyond, encompassing a broad range of developmental challenges. I encountered many children who presented with an as yet unidentified or misunderstood communication difficulty, a developmental delay, an idiosyncratic personality, an emotional disturbance, and so on, who had been labeled elsewhere with this diagnostic alternative as if it were a diagnostic certainty.

A brief personal aside: during many years of clinical work with children, in my reports I never applied PDD or PDD-NOS as a diagnosis of a child. I tacitly refused to apply a diagnostic term which I felt did not provide me with diagnostic clarity. This does not mean that I denied that a particular child was suffering from a developmental difficulty. The challenge was always to use interactive play and/or play-based cognitive tasks to elucidate more clearly the child's developmental challenges and strengths; to generate hypotheses about the roots of a child's condition; to arrive at a clearer understanding of the child's functional difficulties; to attempt to determine the possible reasons for the child's presentation; to interactively, playfully explore to what degree presenting symptoms were deeply entrenched or could yet prove amenable to positive change; in short, to arrive at a *differential understanding* of each child's weaknesses and strengths in order to design individually suited interventions.

The *DSM-5* and Autism

Perhaps it was an acknowledgment of the interrelated, elastic criteria for autism in the *DSM-IV-TR* that led to the official reconfiguration of the criteria for autism in the *DSM-5* in 2013. Was greater diagnostic clarity achieved? In the *DSM-5*, the clinical categories of Autistic Disorder, Childhood Disintegrative Disorder, Asperger's Disorder and Pervasive Developmental Disorder were eliminated, with Rett's Disorder reclassified as a neurological disorder of genetic origin and removed from this grouping. Instead, all of these disorders were melded and amalgamated into one vast "spectrum," Autistic Spectrum Disorder (ASD), which appears under the global heading of Neurodevelopmental Disorders.

The official *DSM-5* diagnostic criteria for ASD are organized in only two categories, as opposed to the three categories of the *DSM-IV-TR*. These categories are:

• Persistent deficits in social communication and social interaction across settings.
• Restricted, repetitive patterns of behavior, interests or activities.

Omitted from the *DSM-5* criteria is "a delay in or total lack of the development of spoken language," as appeared in the *DSM-IV-TR*. The *DSM-5* autism criteria appear to stress the more social aspects rather than the linguistic aspects of communication. This absence of a reference to "a lack of spoken language" within the *DSM-5* autism criteria is puzzling and a concern. Historically, among the eleven foundational cases with which Kanner introduced his clinical configuration of autism, those children presented with a range of verbal communication impairments, ranging from a mute, nonverbal presentation to verbal idiosyncrasies, aberrations and deficits.[5] According to Kanner's descriptions, common among these children was the fact that some degree of verbal impairment was thought to typify an autistic presentation, even though Kanner considered verbal impairments a "secondary" characteristic, following his "primary characteristics" of emotional aloneness and perseverative behavior.[6] So verbal impairments, even if secondary, were significant in the original criteria for diagnosing autism.

The omission of a criterion related to a lack of spoken language opens the door for the inclusion into the ASD category of children (and adults) who possess spoken language yet who may now find themselves at risk of being diagnosed or misdiagnosed as autistic. In short, the current *DSM-5* array of ASD symptoms has expanded significantly from Kanner's initial succinct formulation of an autistic condition—unfortunately though, in a worryingly generalized direction.

In the *DSM-5*, the first cluster of diagnostic criteria for ASD, deficits in social communication and social interaction, comprises three subsets of symptoms (paraphrased here with italics added):

- Deficits in social-emotional reciprocity, *ranging*, for example, from abnormal social approach and failure of normal back-and-forth conversation to reduced sharing of interests, emotions or affect, to failure to initiate or respond to social interactions.
- Deficits in nonverbal communicative behaviors used for social interaction, *ranging*, for example, from poorly integrated verbal and nonverbal communication to abnormalities in eye contact and body language or deficits in understanding and use of gestures, to a total lack of facial expressions and nonverbal communication.
- Deficits in developing, maintaining and understanding relationships, *ranging*, for example, from difficulties adjusting behavior to suit various social contexts to difficulties in sharing imaginative play or in making friends; to absence of interest in peers.

The second cluster of ASD diagnostic criteria relates to restricted, repetitive patterns of behavior, interests or activities, as manifested by at least two of the following:

- Stereotyped or repetitive motor movements, use of objects or speech.
- Insistence on sameness; inflexible adherence to routines or ritualized patterns of verbal or nonverbal behavior.
- Highly restricted, fixated interests, abnormal in intensity or focus.

- Hyper- or hyporeactivity to sensory input or unusual interest in sensory aspects of the environment.

Putting a few of these key phrases under our magnifying glass, we note the extent of the various ranges in the first symptom grouping: from an abnormal social approach . . . to failure to initiate social interaction; from poorly integrated verbal and nonverbal communication . . . to abnormalities in eye contact and body language . . . to a lack of . . . nonverbal communication; from difficulties adjusting behavior to suit social contexts . . . to difficulties in sharing imaginative play.

How can clinical specificity or a reliable differential diagnosis be achieved if we are using criteria that present us with a *range* of symptom options? Also, the ranges of behaviors are vast and expansive. A child with oral dyspraxia (like Max, Chapter 7), or emotional disturbances (like Annie or Josh, Chapters 3 and 8), or selective mutism, or certain genetic deficits, or a traumatized child, or a language-delayed typical child (like Davie, Chapter 4)—all could easily present within these "ranges."

The result is serious diagnostic uncertainty. While there may well be other environmental, brain function and/or genetic reasons that account for the proliferation of the autism diagnosis today, I worry that the broadly configured criteria for AD and PDD-NOS (formerly) and for ASD (currently) account for no small part of the "epidemic of autism" one hears about so often. Also, as discussed above, the elastic spectrum criteria of the *DSM-5* now encompass "verbal" children who may also have other features typical of the ASD diagnosis. Surely these factors would virtually guarantee an exponential proliferation of that diagnosis.

One further observation relevant to both the *DSM-IV-TR* and the *DSM-5*: the group of symptoms that pertain to stereotypical behavior does echo one of the benchmarks of the autistic condition defined by Kanner.[7] The symptoms related to perseverative stereotypical behaviors (when accompanied by extreme emotional cutoffness) come closest to signaling Kanner's conceptualization of a genuine autistic condition—but with one critical proviso. One must be careful to avoid the kind of faulty logic often observed in the field—that of mistaking a particular behavioral manifestation as sure proof of the general autism diagnosis.

To clarify: it is true that a genuinely autistic child (using a stringent interpretation of Kanner's criteria) usually engages in such perseverative behaviors as hand-flapping, rocking or walking in certain circuits. However, in dynamically assessing children, I saw that *not every child* who engages in hand-flapping or who insists on a particular route to preschool is necessarily autistic. Similarly, it is true that a genuinely autistic child will be preoccupied with repetitive, perseverative types of play, such as lining up blocks or cars. However, it is not true that *any child* who strictly arrays blocks or cars is necessarily autistic. Careful clinical discernment, an internalization of Kanner's more restricted primary criteria for autism and, above all, the willingness to actively engage and attempt to seek strengths and to modify presenting symptoms—all these will help the practitioner determine whether one is looking at genuine autism or a developmental condition that appears on the surface to be autism, yet is not.

Finally, the *DSM-5* text regarding the ASD diagnosis cautions that the symptoms must be present early in life, yet the text states that older individuals whose social difficulties may be masked by "learned strategies" in later life may also be included in this category. The boundaries of what was once considered a developmental condition of early childhood (cf. pervasive *developmental* disorder) have been expanded to include older individuals.

There are a few diagnostic provisos. The *DSM-5* text specifies that the symptoms must also cause clinically significant impairment in varied areas of current functioning. Also, the practitioner should note whether there is or is not accompanying intellectual impairment, language impairment and/or a genetic or medical condition.

A subsequent table, not reproduced in Appendix II, reflects the attempt within the *DSM-5* to consider the severity of symptoms: severe, marked or moderate. The severity levels are assessed descriptively according to the degree of impaired function the deficit causes, along with a consideration as to whether the child's condition requires "very substantial support," "substantial support" or simply "support." But do these delineations of "required support" actually shed light on the severity of the autistic condition or, rather, reflect other subjective, interrelated factors? For example, might not the perception of "severe" symptoms be influenced by the level of the practitioner's ease, comfort and facility in engaging and modifying the symptoms? A skilled, creative therapist might conclude that a child requires only moderate support. An institution with severe staff and budgetary constraints might conclude that the same child requires intense support. Wouldn't a parent who is overwhelmed by having a child with even mild special needs perceive and describe that child's needs for support as severe? Similarly, a child with mild social communication problems, who under better bureaucratic circumstances might be a superior candidate for educational inclusion, could be perceived as requiring "very substantial support," if that child happens to be placed in a school with a reluctant or inadequate policy of educational inclusion.

Multiple Roots for Single Behaviors

An underlying conceptual difficulty with the autism criteria of the former *DSM-IV-TR* and the current *DSM-5* is the focus on phenomena observable in the behavioral realm. This point was raised earlier in this chapter, but it deserves further attention. When using the *DSM-IV-TR*, the practitioner noted that the child was not pointing, or could not initiate or sustain a conversation. With the *DSM-5*, and the shift to noting behaviors which fall within an extensive "range," there is even less clarity, but there is still an attempt to focus the practitioner on observable behaviors, such as "difficulties in sharing imaginative play," "rigid thinking patterns" or "adverse response to specific sounds or textures."

One might argue: "So what is the problem? Obviously, we must substantiate our clinical reasoning with observable data!" But there is a problem here. Behaviors have a vast array of reasons, motives, emotional nuances and colorations, environmentally influenced reasons and roots. Beneath the surface of each observable behavior lie multifaceted worlds.

Consider, for example, a child who is not speaking, isolating himself within the classroom and avoiding peers on the playground: perhaps the child is autistic. But, he or she might be suffering from selective mutism, from a speech defect which causes embarrassment, from an undiagnosed hearing problem, from the traumatic impact of physical or sexual abuse, from a profound lack of confidence due to emotional distress and so on. Consider as well children who exhibit extreme reactions to sensory stimuli: they may fall under the rubric of autism. Or, they may be suffering from sensory overload (like Josh, Chapter 8) and in need of coping and desensitizing strategies, with their conditions completely unrelated to any autistic nuance. Similarly, children with perseverative behaviors like hand-flapping may be autistic. Or, their repetitive behaviors may be related to sensory overload, neurological immaturity or complications, or extreme anxiety, with no need to place the child within an autistic "range" of behaviors and thus saddle the child with the risk of a falsely positive autism-related diagnosis. The focus on observable behaviors associated with autism, without comprehensive attention to the underlying physiological, emotional and contextual roots of these behaviors, risks tipping the scales toward the misdiagnosis or overuse of the term autism.

In less frequent situations where symptom checklists[8] had been used elsewhere to diagnose the child, my parallel goal was to help parents understand that a single behavioral symptom has many varied roots. From the Feuerstein perspective, a tallying of symptoms can only remain a superficial summation without a dynamic, qualitative understanding and active encounter with each symptom and a parallel search for strengths. Even when symptom lists had been used to ascertain an ASD diagnosis, my goal was to help parents think clearly and critically about the implications of the tallied numbers that account for the visible above ground, but do not attend to the myriad possible roots, causes and nuances of that behavior.

In a minority of cases, the relatively recent ADOS[9] had been used to determine the child's autism diagnosis.[10] While the ADOS enjoys much positive regard because of its central interactive play component and attendant extensive parent interview, there were occasions when I discovered that by seeking the child behind the symptoms and discerning islets of normalcy, my conclusion contradicted that of the professional who had arrived at an ASD diagnosis using the ADOS. The intention here is not to cast aspersions on this instrument, but to suggest that working dynamically, interactively and with an emphasis on qualitative description, probing the malleability of symptoms while seeking strengths—islets of normalcy—has the power to reach behind evident symptoms, and to create a more positive diagnostic and prognostic picture.

A final point for reflection: the *DSM* presents no information regarding the consideration of a suspected autistic child's strengths and ability to change, as the Feuerstein paradigm tenaciously advocates. It is as if the granting of an autistic spectrum diagnosis explains all and summarizes the child's identity. Sadly, this often predetermines the child's anticipated developmental trajectory. A sum total of symptoms does not take into account their degree of modifiability.

Then What Did They Have?

A parent or practitioner reading this book may be inclined to respond that surely practitioners would distinguish between autistic-like symptoms rooted in underconfidence, mutism, emotional disturbance or a hearing impairment from a condition of autism. Many do. Yet the stories of the children in this book argue that autism misdiagnoses are rife and easily attained. A central difficulty, as this discussion has suggested, appears to lie with the broadly configured formal autism criteria. These elastic criteria enable alternative explanations for a child's situation to fall too readily into the category of an autism-related diagnosis. It is not farfetched to say that there is a high probability that a conscientious practitioner using this elastic diagnostic yardstick with a child who presents with any of a range of social communication problems coupled with behavioral idiosyncrasies will arrive at a "spectrum" diagnosis.

When lecturing to parents, students or practitioners, I was often asked, "Well, if those children weren't autistic, then what were they? What did they have?" These questions themselves reflect a reigning mindset that if we don't give a condition/situation a specific diagnostic label then we haven't done our clinical jobs. Naturally, there is also pressure from public and private insurance interests to codify and therefore pigeonhole a child's condition. In order to reach the child behind the symptoms, we need to do much more than determine a diagnosis. We need to arrive at an understanding of the child's presentation. When considering autism, using listed criteria to arrive at a specific diagnosis as opposed to probing the roots, ramifications and strategies for the amelioration of a child's difficulties are not equivalent. For many of the children diagnosed previously as autistic, whom I later encountered in my office and found to possess normative or near-normative faculties, the overgenerous use of the elastic terminology of an official autism diagnosis was not conjecture. It was a fact.

Responding to the query "If they weren't autistic, then what were they?" I present here a listing of several of the underlying and often previously undetected difficulties which had been masked by an autism diagnosis among those children I assessed and treated. A brief annotation of these as encountered in my clinical work follows.

Mutism. Children with selective mutism are usually identifiable by the contrasting environments in which they are or are not prepared to speak. Sometimes, however, I encountered seriously underconfident, quiet, verbally impaired or emotionally disturbed children, whose "virtual mutism," as one might call it, had been misinterpreted by a practitioner and then mis-diagnosed as "spectrum."

Rett's Disorder. Throughout my career, I encountered a small number of girls in whom I suspected this rare genetic syndrome. Their Rett's Disorder had not yet been identified, and they had been diagnosed elsewhere as autistic. In those cases not yet identified as Rett's, certain motor idiosyncrasies in the children caught my attention. I then tactfully encouraged the parents to consult with a pediatric neurologist to explore several conditions, suggesting that a neurologist or a geneticist rule out Rett's Disorder as well. The actual diagnosis of Rett's, if applicable, was then carried out by a medical expert.

Mild to moderate emotional disturbances or more extreme disturbances such as pre-, post-, borderline- and psychotic conditions. Beyond moderate emotional disturbances, there were a small number of children whose emotional overload was so extreme that it had pushed them beyond contact with self and with reality. Their behaviors reflected the deeper emotional disturbance of a psychotic condition. For a number of these children, their peculiar behaviors and idiosyncratic style of social communication had resulted in an erroneous autism diagnosis, with the underlying emotional disturbances often left un-treated under the presumption that autism was the problem. Professor Feuerstein's understanding of psychiatric conditions was invaluable in helping to distinguish children's presentations related to psychosis.

Moderate to profound hearing impairments. One might be tempted to assume that the detection of hearing impairments would be a given in assessing a child with a developmental challenge related to communication. Unfortunately, I found that this was not always the case. I often encountered young children with mild to moderate hearing impairments, usually caused by chronic ear infections and fluids, who had been misdiagnosed as autistic (such as Davie, Chapter 4). The assessing practitioner had apparently taken the child's "lack of social communication" at face value and had not considered sending the child to a specialist for a hearing test. Alternatively, there were a number of children whose hearing deficits had been clearly identified but whose ac-companying behaviors and social problems had been misinterpreted as being a function of autism, rather than a logical outgrowth of the isolation that a hearing impairment induces (such as Amy, Chapter 12). If not properly equipped with signing or lip-reading skills, or more currently a cochlear im-plant, deaf or seriously hearing-impaired children, I observed, were at risk of a falsely positive "autistic" diagnosis. Energetically eliciting signs of emotional responsiveness, intellectual comprehension, reciprocity and humor helped me ascertain whether the child's degree of social communication dysfunction was entrenched in the emotional isolation and aloneness of autism, or was a result of a sense of cutoffness that can accompany serious hearing difficulties. If, through play interaction, I observed that qualities reflecting warmth and a sense of emotional connection were present despite problems with speech acquisition, often it was possible to safely negate the misdiagnosis of autism, prioritize the hearing deficit and adjust treatment plans accordingly.

Brain abnormalities and genetic syndromes. Parents' accounts and the medical information accompanying a referral often cited specific brain abnormalities or a specific genetic syndrome along with the suspected autism diagnosis (comorbidity). In many cases, the autism diagnosis appeared to have over-ridden the underlying physiological difficulty, and treatment recommendations had been made, sometimes erroneously, based more on the presumed autism than on the impact of the underlying physiological problems.

Oral dyspraxia. A child with oral dyspraxia experiences, to various degrees, difficulties with brain messages to the many muscles of tongue, lips and jaw that are necessary for clear speech production. While there may well be children with oral dyspraxia who are genuinely autistic, not all children who are orally dyspraxic are necessarily autistic. I encountered quite a few (like Max, Chapter 7) whose undeniable difficulty in speech production and sub-sequent social communication problems had been misinterpreted and mis-diagnosed as PDD-NOS or ASD.

Children with "garden variety" developmental difficulties. Sometimes the underlying or compounding developmental difficulty of a child is discernible or detectable through medical evaluation: a genetic syndrome, a hearing loss, an identified brain abnormality, a specific emotional or physical trauma. However, I often encountered children whose developmental difficulties seemed to fall between the cracks. All of the medical, genetic and neurological tests had yielded normal results. There was no definitive cause that could be pinpointed for the child's developmental glitch, and yet it was clear that something was not quite right.

While children with various developmental problems may indeed be autistic, not all children with miscellaneous developmental problems are necessarily autistic. Yet they are at great risk for being misdiagnosed as autistic. Such children often present as "atypical" and "unusual" in some regard. Perhaps it is this quality about their presentation that garnered them a place in the elastic and overly-inclusive PDD or "spectrum" diagnoses.

Typical children with developmental delays. In this casebook, Jack, Sasha, Annie, Davie, Max and Josh are representative of the many children I saw with normal abilities yet whose presenting difficulties had elsewhere resulted in an autism-related diagnosis. Their subsequent development revealed their latent normative capabilities. The reasons for their initially worrisome presentations varied: language delay, emotional overload, extreme sensory sensitivities or just the need for a little more time to mature. It was always gratifying to nurture the children with normative inner potential behind the symptoms which had been mistaken for autism. At the same time, it was distressing to comprehend the ease with which the autism diagnosis had been attached to these children initially.

An important caution, in particular to parents: the above listing *does not in any way imply or suggest* that if your child is not genuinely autistic then he or she necessarily suffers from any of the above conditions. The above section is a general report from the field, a summary of the most typical kinds of errors I observed in the misdiagnoses of young children suspected to have autism. This list should *in no way* be considered predictive or descriptive of your own child. Arriving at an alternative understanding of a child's underlying difficulty which had become obscured by a diagnosis of autism usually required hours of patient observation, interviews with parents, a careful review of the medical history and, of course, active and energetic interaction with a child to determine the entrenchment versus the modifiability of a child's symptoms. A comprehensive clinical look at each child rather than a listing of his or her behavioral symptoms led to the above alternative clinical understanding of the children's presentations.

What Does the "D" for Disorder Mean for Autism?

There is one additional underlying difficulty to be probed in our close reading of the formal autism criteria: what, after all, is a disorder? The introductory material of the *DSM-IV-TR* placed the notion of "disorder" squarely in the realm of "mental disorder" and admitted frankly that ascertaining the definition of a mental disorder was a challenge in many respects. The text grappled first of all with the fact that the term mental disorder implies a mind-body distinction. The text goes on to acknowledge that this is a distinction which is no longer adhered to, since current research and practice have revealed the intricate interconnection between the realms of mind and body. The text also acknowledged that finding a "consistent operational definition [for mental disorder], one that would cover all situations and contexts, could not really be ascertained."[11] The introductory text concluded that the process of *identifying the problems in defining* "mental disorder" was much easier than *finding a solution for an accurate definition.* Following these caveats, the text frankly admits that the ensuing definition of a mental disorder was, essentially, as "useful as any other." Finally, the following definition of a mental disorder is offered: "a clinically significant behavioral syndrome or pattern that is associated with distress or disability."[12]

Like the earlier *DSM IV-TR*, the introductory discussion of the *DSM-5* similarly states that no definition of "disorder" can satisfactorily capture all aspects of all disorders. Refraining from itemizing the caveats of the *DSM-IV-TR*, the *DSM-5* defines a mental disorder as a "syndrome characterized by significant disturbance in an individual's cognition, emotional regulation, or behavior and which reflects a dysfunction in the psychological, biological, or developmental processes underlying mental functioning."[13]

Where does the notion of "mental disorder" leave us in relation to the conceptualization of autism in young children? With many questions—whose putative answers have serious implications as to how we view the potential modifiability of the child who presents with autistiform symptoms. Does the inclusion of autism diagnostic criteria within a manual of psychiatric diagnoses imply that autism is a psychiatric condition? Years ago Kanner assumed so, and he concluded that childhood or infantile autism was an offshoot or subset of psychotic or childhood schizophrenic conditions, a conceptualization that, to the best of my knowledge, no longer reigns.[14]

The term "mental disorder" appears to be closely associated in the *DSM* with the word "syndrome." Does this mean that autism is inherently genetic, like Down syndrome? A syndrome also has medical research connotations. Does this mean that "autism" is a kind of developmental disease? I often met practitioners who appeared to regard autism as if it were an incurable condition or a developmental disease. Should a term like *mental* disorder, with all its connotations of disturbance, apply to autism, which is a *developmental* challenge? Children develop. Children can change. Should the notion of a syndrome or a disorder, with all the finality these terms imply, attach to young children who are often significantly modifiable to the extent that the autism diagnosis may no longer apply to them a few years later?

As the reader might have deduced, deep in the trenches of the actual work with the children, I did not devote too much time to unraveling detailed answers to these important conceptual questions, because the challenge of catalyzing meaningful changes within the children's presentations was too great and too exciting. My colleagues and I, inspired by Feuerstein's work in human modifiability, steered clear of any conceptualization of autism—such as disorder, syndrome or disease—that foreclosed hope or inhibited the possibility of our eliciting change within a child.

Over the years I learned to be comfortable with putting a suspected autism diagnosis aside and with adopting as a baseline for assessment the simple understanding that the child is presenting with a generic "social communication problem." However, I then expected from myself to get to know and to try to understand the child deeply, to probe the answers to dozens of questions related to childhood realities, the family constellation and relationships, physiological and/or sensory deficits, birth trauma and developmental blocks, the degree of environmental linguistic richness and many other factors to help me understand, qualitatively, functionally, empathically, the operative roots of a child's social communication problem.

Anxious or even grieving parents whose child had been diagnosed as AD, PDD-NOS or ASD were often surprised when they read the broad and all-encompassing official diagnostic criteria. Glimpsing a "behind-the-scenes" insight into the nuts and bolts of hyperelastic and overgenerously configured diagnostic criteria often gave distressed parents both hope and strength—hope that their child was not truly autistic according to Kanner's essential primary criteria, and strength to find the right therapies and strategies to help their child develop according to his or her own more precisely understood individual needs. The parents of nearly all of the children represented in this casebook felt strengthened when they began to understand the elasticity of the formal autism diagnostic criteria, although some continued to wrestle with doubts about the accuracy of the diagnosis for years, until their children's normative or near normative progress during early school years ultimately proved reassuring.

Too often the diagnosis of autism does not illumine our understanding of a child. Rather, the rubric of a PDD, AD or ASD diagnosis *masks* our understanding of the child and then confounds the treatment planning. If a child with virtually *any* kind of social communication problem is at risk of being labeled autistic, as my experience taught, then I worry that the field has essentially given up on the art of differential diagnosis with this population. If not a differential *diagnosis*, then certainly a differential *understanding* of each child with a communication problem is possible—and necessary. Do we fail as practitioners if we cannot give a child's presentation a specific name and code? I think not. I think we risk failure when in our rush to label or code we miss the complex interaction of dynamics that burden each child who presents with whatever combination of social/communication/perseveration difficulties. It is our depth of understanding, our search for a differential comprehension of each child, not the diagnosis, which should inform and guide our assessment process and our treatment interventions.

In the familiar tale of the emperor who parades in the street wearing nothing, all of the king's subjects listen to the proclamation that the emperor has new clothes and allow the verbal proclamation to override what they see. The king is persuaded by his tailor and his aides that he is actually wearing fine attire. His many subjects, influenced by the royal proclamation of new clothes, appear in awe of the king's lovely "new clothes." The rubric of "new clothes" and the presumption of what "must be" cloud their vision—except, of course, for one young subject who sees what is.

What we call something can determine what we allow ourselves to see. There are parents and practitioners who do see beneath the veil of what has become a too broadly configured diagnostic term. They are looking for signs of the real and responsive child behind the autistiform symptoms.

Notes

1 American Psychiatric Association, *Diagnostic and Statistical Manual of Mental Disorders: DSM IV-TR* (Arlington, VA: American Psychiatric Association, 2000).

2 American Psychiatric Association, *Diagnostic and Statistical Manual of Mental Disorders: DSM-5* (Arlington, VA: American Psychiatric Association, 2013).

3 American Psychiatric Association, *Diagnostic and Statistical Manual of Mental Disorders: DSM-I* (Arlington, VA: American Psychiatric Association, 1952).

4 Leo Kanner, *Childhood Psychosis: Initial Studies and New Insights* (Washington, DC: Winston, 1973).

5 Ibid.

6 Ibid.

7 Ibid.

8 David A. Krug, Joel R. Arick, and Patricia Almond, "Autism Behavior Checklist-ABC," in *ASIEP-3* (Torrance, CA: Western Psychological Services, 2008); Diana

Robins, Deborah Fein, and Marianne Barton, "The Modified Checklist of Autism in Toddlers, Revised with Follow-up" (M-CHAT-R/F) (Author copyright, 2009); Eric Schopler et al., *Childhood Autism Rating Scale, Second Edition (CARS-2): For Diagnostic Screening and Classification of Autism* (Torrance, CA: Western Psychological Services, 2010). The ABC, the CARS-2 and the parent-completed M-CHAT-R/F are symptom checklists commonly used as part of a comprehensive evaluation of autism. Interestingly, in my work in Israel, I encountered very few children for whom these instruments had been a part of the autism evaluation the children underwent before arriving at the Institute. Nearly all had been diagnosed using the *DSM*.

9 Catherine Lord et al., *Autism Diagnostic Observation Schedule, ADOS-2* (Torrance, CA: Western Psychological Services, 2012).

10 For reasons unclear to me, only a small minority of Israeli practitioners whose reports I received had used the ADOS to ascertain the autism diagnosis. Most had used the *DSM* criteria.

11 American Psychiatric Association, *Diagnostic and Statistical Manual of Mental Disorders: DSM-IV-TR* (Arlington, VA: American Psychiatric Association, 2000), xxi.

12 Ibid.

13 American Psychiatric Association, *Diagnostic and Statistical Manual of Mental Disorders: DSM-5* (Arlington, VA: American Psychiatric Association, 2013), 20.

14 Kanner, *Childhood Psychosis.*

References

American Psychiatric Association. *Diagnostic and Statistical Manual of Mental Disorders: DSM-I.* Arlington, VA: American Psychiatric Association, 1952.

American Psychiatric Association. *Diagnostic and Statistical Manual of Mental Disorders: DSM-IV-TR.* Arlington, VA: American Psychiatric Association, 2000.

American Psychiatric Association. *Diagnostic and Statistical Manual of Mental Disorders: DSM-5.* Arlington, VA: American Psychiatric Association, 2013.

Kanner, Leo. *Childhood Psychosis: Initial Studies and New Insights.* Washington, DC: Winston, 1973.

Krug, David A., Joel R. Arick, and Patricia Almond. "Autism Behavior Checklist-ABC." In *ASIEP-3.* Torrance, CA: Western Psychological Services, 2008.

Lord, Catherine, Michael Rutter, Pamela C. Dilavore, Susan Risi, Katherine Gotham, and Somer L. Bishop. *Autism Diagnostic Observation Schedule, ADOS-2.* Torrance, CA: Western Psychological Services, 2012.

Robins, Diana, Deborah Fein, and Marianne Barton. "The Modified Checklist of Autism in Toddlers, Revised with Follow-up, M-CHAT-R/F." Author copyright, 2009.

Schopler, Eric, Mary E. Van Bourgondian, Glenna J. Wellman, and Steven R. Rose. *Childhood Autism Rating Scale, Second Edition (CARS-2): For Diagnostic Screening and Classification of Autism.* Torrance, CA: Western Psychological Services, 2010.

14 Autistiform but Not Autistic

If the expansively elastic autism criteria of the former *DSM-IV-TR* and the current *DSM-5* do not offer the solace of diagnostic specificity, as the previous chapter suggested, how might we better consider children who present with varying degrees of social communication challenges and perseverative features in a way which keeps their developmental options open?

At the Feuerstein Institute, the answer to this question was: by actually putting the diagnosis aside; by paying careful attention to the details of a child's strengths (islets of normalcy) despite their evident developmental difficulties; by focusing attention on the child's process of change and transformation rather measuring the child's performance on discrete tasks; and by providing in our reports rich descriptions of the overall developmental picture rather than labeling the child with an autism diagnosis, if we were convinced that it was not applicable.

Interestingly, the number of children whom I saw over the years who presented with genuine autism according to a stringent interpretation of Kanner's criteria—emotionally cut off and unreachable to an extreme degree, lacking communicative interest and facility, as well as obsessively preoccupied with perseverative behaviors such as hand-flapping or rocking—was extremely small: twenty, thirty perhaps, out of the many hundreds whom my colleagues and I saw who had received an autism-related diagnosis elsewhere. Even with children who evidenced the most extreme presentations, we proceeded as above: seeking glimmers of non-symptomatic behavior to use as a fragile toehold from which to generate further change; seeking evidence of modifiability across assessment and treatment sessions; and by using our reports as educational tools to share with parents and practitioners our interpretation of the child's symptoms and our proposed strategies for meaningfully assisting the child.

Jack, Sasha, Annie, Davie, Max and Josh were not autistic. What were they? And so, to return to the question posed at the beginning of this chapter, what diagnosis did we use for children who presented with symptoms that appeared to be autistic but whose dynamic assessments revealed that their profile did not fit that of classical Kanner autism? The short answer is: at the Feuerstein Institute we did not necessarily seek another diagnosis for the child. We sought to *understand* each child's developmental predicament and to generate a profile of modifiability. At times the dynamic work led to another more accurate diagnostic label for the child, particularly when we perceived physiological complications that required the child's referral to a medical specialist. However, most often with children experiencing developmental difficulties, we avoided the temptation to seek a "closest fit" diagnosis. We preferred to understand the complexity of the child's difficulties, prioritize strengths, and create viable recommendations as a basis for a program of change.

Over the years, I occasionally met other professionals who, like the Feuerstein staff, preferred not to pigeonhole a child in the autism category when their assessment and treatment of the child was demonstrating that the child was well on the way to leaving his or her autistic-like symptoms behind. In seeking an accurate, relevant diagnosis that would not confine the child for years to an autism diagnosis, some of these other practitioners selected another aspect of the child's presentation on which to focus their diagnosis, preferring to attach to the child a diagnosis that pertained to a more transient condition and a diagnosis that imparts less stigma and fewer preconceptions about the child than autism often does. For example, if anxiety was a relevant feature in the presentation of a child who had social communication difficulties but who also evidenced excellent developmental potential, one practitioner mentioned that she preferred to prioritize the anxiety in the child's profile and to diagnose the child as suffering from an Anxiety Disorder. If genuine autism proved to be a fact in that child's life in the future, naturally she would revise the diagnosis accordingly.

For most of the many hundreds of children diagnosed as autistic before their arrival at the Institute, a more appropriate description of their symptoms—useful precisely because it is *not* a diagnosis—would have been "autistiform," a term I found most helpful in conceptualizing a child's presentation. "Autistiform" is a term which has been in clinical use for years but which, I believe, is deserving of more widespread usage. It should be taken out of dusty drawers, polished and elevated to a sparkling status and useful function in distinguishing the symptoms of children who only appear to be autistic from those with acknowledged extreme presentations who truly are.

Autistiform means just that: behaviors which have the surface appearance, the form but not necessarily the essence, of autism. Autistiform suggests "kind of autistic," "sort of autistic," "autistic-like," "reminds me of autism." But it does not necessarily mean that the child is emotionally cut off, obsessively perseverative and unreachable. The child's symptoms *appear* to be those characteristic of autism. Autistiform behaviors recall autism, but at the same time a term like autistiform behaviors, symptoms or features leaves the door open for healthy doubt and creative options for realizing that the child's initial presentation may be modifiable to a significant degree. Reinvigorating the usage of the term autistiform symptoms would go a long way toward reminding parents and practitioners that a child who appears autistic may not actually be so.

When lecturing to parents, educators or practitioners, I often enjoyed explaining the difference between the terms *autistic* and *autistiform* by using a classic chicken soup example. Perhaps you recall grandma's wonderful, richly fragrant chicken soup with dumplings and carrots floating in the delicious broth? Real chicken soup! Now compare that with your canned or packaged variety. It looks like chicken soup, and it smells something like it, but it is certainly lacking the essence of the real thing. Metaphorically, that is the difference between autistic and autistiform.

Currently, the prevalence of the term "autistic spectrum disorder" or sometimes even just "spectrum," as if that explains the child's situation, and the elastic criteria of the (former) *DSM-IV* and the *DSM-5* blur the critical differences between genuine autism and approximations of autism. My experience taught that it is far too easy for a child who "looks as if" he or she is autistic to be formally diagnosed as truly autistic. This book offers testimony to the prevalence of the misdiagnosis of autistiform behavior and to the fact that a condition that appears at first glance to be autism may not be so at all.

If the *DSM* autism criteria are so elastic and the term autistiform is also general, what then are the advantages of using the term "autistiform" to describe the symptoms instead of "spectrum" to diagnose the child? When we hear a medical diagnosis, we like to feel that we are standing on the bedrock of science, of clear-cut, research-grounded knowledge. But, as the previous chapter suggested, the use of the term "spectrum" has essentially dissolved the specificity of a differential diagnosis: if a child *appears* autistic, my experience taught, he or she is at risk of being diagnosed as autistic, whether accurately or not.

In the Introduction, I asked the question: why replace one general term, autistic, with another general concept, autistiform? Precisely because the word "autistiform" is not a diagnosis. "Autistiform" safely describes an impression about a constellation of behaviors. It does not presume to definitively classify the child. It leaves room for the consideration of other factors which may underlie the complexity of each child's condition. Once the official diagnosis of "autistic spectrum" is used, the child's situation is considered to have been determined. All that we know, understand, believe and presume about genuine autism comes into play, and rather than illuminating each child's condition, the over-generous diagnosis actually obscures the intricacies of each child who "appears autistic."

The term autistiform is advantageous because it intrinsically reminds and cautions practitioners and parents that initially we are dealing with "forms," with surface appearances. Using the term autistiform is clinically helpful precisely because it is not a diagnosis or a substitute diagnosis. It leaves open the options for our clinical understanding. As noted, it is a general descriptor of symptoms which keeps alive and uppermost in mind a healthy doubt about the presence of genuine autism. The term challenges us as practitioners to probe beneath the symptoms, to explore the child's hidden strengths, and to determine the modifiability of symptoms which may at first appear to be intransigent, impenetrable.

To summarize the essentials: it is true that a child may present with a combination of behaviors typical of autism and, indeed, be genuinely autistic. But, as these casebook stories illustrate, it is all too possible that a child exhibiting such behaviors is not genuinely autistic at all. He or she may appear autistic, with behaviors merely autisti*form*. They have the form, the outward semblance of autism, but they lack the substance of a truly autistic condition, rooted in Kanner's original perception of emotional aloneness, cutoffness, and obsession with perseveration.

Annie (Chapter 3) initially appeared cut off, but she proved reachable and she later changed profoundly. Josh (Chapter 8) presented as anxiously silent and avoidant, yet several years later he was a successful, outgoing, socially popular student. Sammy's communication (Chapter 10) at first appeared totally blocked, but he later displayed a warm, expressive personality. The term autistiform would have offered a more appropriate description of the initial presentations of nearly all the children in this book, and many more whom I saw as well.

It is an intriguing fact that most of the children in this casebook had received an autism-related diagnosis despite the fact that nearly all of them *did not evidence* any stereotypical behaviors such as hand-flapping, object-waving, circuit-walking or rocking. What does this mean? For Sasha, Annie, Davie, Max, Josh, Gordie and others, we can assume that this means that these children had *appeared* to other professionals to be autistic because of their verbal and social communication problems. The lack of obsessively perseverative behaviors, a key facet of genuine autism, had been overlooked by practitioners, perhaps because of the uniqueness of the children's social communication challenges. The children's presentations had been unusual, idiosyncratic, perhaps even difficult to classify, but all had in common some kind of social communication difficulty. Even though they lacked perseverative behaviors, they had *appeared* to other practitioners as autistic, a fact that had led too quickly to an autism diagnosis. The "autistiform" descriptor for their symptoms would have been more apt.

Does it matter that very few of the children whom I assessed were genuinely autistic, as delineated by Kanner's primary criteria, even though the referral information claimed that they were? It matters very much if a falsely positive formal diagnosis of autism or ASD is used as the basis for treatment and educational placement decisions. If, however, a child's unique individual needs, weaknesses, challenges and especially strengths and potential for modification, rather than a diagnosis, are used as the basis for treatment and educational decisions, our clinical work will be so much sounder. Using the term autistiform, not as a diagnosis but simply as a guiding descriptor of symptoms, reminds us that when working in the realm of child development, it is important to energetically seek the emotional/developmental content beneath the form, the real child behind the autistiform symptoms.

15 Toward a Paradigm Shift

Searching for the child behind the autistiform symptoms entails embarking on a paradigm shift for many parents and practitioners, away from a symptom focus and toward a holistic, functional appreciation and understanding of the child. When one begins to internalize the practical, functional wisdom, individual attunement and the positive clinical potential of the qualitative dynamic approach to assessment, adopts interactive play techniques as a basis for assessment and treatment of the young child with autistiform features and uses a dynamic rather than a conventional perspective as the basis for recommendations, such a paradigm shift can literally yield life-saving results, as the story of Ben, interwoven throughout this chapter, will illustrate.

Introducing Ben

Ben was five years old when he first arrived at the Institute. He appeared shy and somewhat fearful. His parents appeared stressed and worried. A fair and sensitive child, Ben's expressive language and social interactions lagged behind anticipated abilities for his chronological age. He had recently been seen in several highly-regarded clinics and hospitals, all of which had concluded that Ben had PDD, then the frequently used term for an autistic condition. Various child development specialists, all considered experts in autism, had based their diagnoses on the then applicable *DSM-IV-TR* criteria. All of the specialists had recommended unequivocally that Ben be placed in a special kindergarten for autistic children where, it was assumed, he would benefit from the intensive speech therapy and specialized attention available in such a setting.

Although Ben's assessment and follow-up sojourn at the Institute were relatively short, just over eighteen months, the use of the dynamic approach advocated by Feuerstein in assessing him and in formulating recommendations to his parents impacted on the entire trajectory of his development, into adulthood. The case of Ben well illustrates the primary differences between a conventional approach and the dynamic approach in working with children with autistiform features. These differences are evident in the assessment process, the weight given to the autism diagnosis, the assumptions and expectations associated with the diagnosis, assumptions regarding the impact of the presumed cause of the child's problem (etiology), the methods of working with the child and the scope of the practical advice and recommendations given to parents. Many of these points have received attention throughout this casebook, so they will not be unfamiliar to readers. In this chapter, the key differences between a *dynamic* and a *conventional* way of working with children who present with autistiform features are highlighted and summarized.

Differing Approaches to Assessment

In a *conventional assessment* of autism:

- The process of assessment primarily involves a quantitative process, with the focus on identifying and tallying symptoms, the problematic observable behaviors of the child with autistiform features. This is usually accomplished by applying the *DSM* criteria for autism. Many practitioners may also use autism symptom checklists as part of a comprehensive assessment process.[1] These, too, generally involve quantifying the symptoms.
- The focus of most conventional assessment measures is on pathology, with evidence of exceptional behaviors reflecting personality and developmental strengths often overlooked or disregarded.
- My experience taught that the strengths of children who present with severely autistic features are even more likely to be overlooked during conventional assessment because of the complexity and stubbornness of their symptoms. Yet these are the children whose strengths most urgently need to be identified.
- Surmising from the content of the many reports that accompanied the referral material to us, the conventional assessment process of children presenting with autistic features tends to be more observational than interactional. I encountered few reports from other institutions which utilized play interactions in their assessments of children.

A notable exception is the highly-regarded Autism Diagnostic Observation Schedule (ADOS-2),[2] which is based on developmentally attuned modules of play-based interaction with the child with suspected autism. Yet the ADOS, too, is symptom-based rather than strength-based. Evidence of exceptional, normative, non-symptomatic behaviors are overlooked or considered irrelevant when compared with the overall symptom profile. The administration guidelines of the ADOS explicitly caution the examiner:

> When assigning ratings for atypical behaviors ... observed during the ADOS- 2, the focus is on capturing an abnormality if it is present . . . . [F]or many pro-social behaviors, the occurrence of a few good examples

(e.g. of eye contact or vocalizations) does not indicate an absence of abnormality.[3]

So even with this interactive, play-based instrument, the emphasis is on identifying and scoring impairments.

The practitioner working from Feuerstein's *dynamic* perspective still notes the child's developmental difficulties. However, substantiating pathology or quantifying symptoms is not the focus of the assessment process:

- A dynamic assessment is a qualitative, not quantitative, process. The assessor is not seeking to sum symptoms but to arrive at a full description of the child's functioning.
- Beyond observing the child's functioning in key developmental areas—communication and language, level and type of play, cognition and task orientation, fine and gross motricity, personality and emotional accessibility—the practitioner working in dynamic fashion actively and energetically intervenes, interacts and uses imagination, warmth and creativity to engage the child.
- The practitioner working dynamically strives to elicit changes in the child's presentation *during* the assessment sessions. This means striving to create new islets of normalcy even when they are not yet evident.
- The purpose of the assessment is to arrive at what Feuerstein called a "profile of modifiability,"[4] and to generate evidence in real time of the capacity of the child to move beyond his or her presenting difficulties.
- The dynamic practitioner attends to the sensory, play, cognitive or relationship conditions under which symptoms improve and strategizes playful and cognitive (when developmentally appropriate) methods for continuing this initial modification.
- Exceptional behaviors that reflect more normative functioning are prized rather than disregarded, with the aim of understanding the factors and conditions which prompt the child with suspected autism to look, speak, play or act in a more normative fashion. The practitioner seeks much more than symptoms. The most fleeting evidences of normative behavior and communication, islets of normalcy, are significant.
- Across assessment sessions, the practitioner is sensitive to any changes in the proportion of emergent strengths versus presenting difficulties.

An aside about the critical importance of a first dynamic assessment session is relevant here. Clearly important for arriving at an understanding of the child, an initial dynamic assessment session is also critical for the parents of a child with suspected autism, because this session functions as an introduction for parents to a new way of considering their child. As the stories in this casebook reflect, parents of a child with suspected autism are often buffeted to varying degrees by waves of sadness, anxiety, worry, depression and even despair. All too frequently, these parents have heard discouraging, pessimistic diagnoses and prognoses from practitioners who work in a more conventional, symptom-focused manner. We want to give parents the understanding and the tools of a potentially more hopeful paradigm. When changes, new islets of normalcy, are elicited from the child during dynamic assessment, simultaneous sparks of hope and encouragement are often ignited within the parents.

Differing Outlooks on the Diagnosis

Most practitioners feel that they have not done their job if they fail to accurately provide an accepted label for the condition of the child. From our experience in reviewing the referral material of many hundreds of children considered, and too often misdiagnosed, as autistic, it would appear that the goal of finding the diagnostic label is often compromised by a tendency to select a diagnosis which may not necessarily be an exact fit, but rather the closest fit. In the game of horseshoes, "close" is relevant information and worth some points. Given the qualitative diagnostics necessary to assess a child with suspected autism, the "closest fit" approach can lead to clinical error.

In a *conventional* approach:

- Ascertaining the diagnosis is usually the practitioner's clinical goal when assessing the child.
- A diagnosis of autism is presumed to clarify the child's situation, creating the basis for future intervention decisions, much as a diagnosis usually does in the field of medicine.
- There appears to be strong determinant power given to the diagnoses of autism, whether the former AD and PDD or the current ASD, with many negative and discouraging assumptions about the child's ability to change commonly attached to these diagnoses.

In assisting distressed parents regarding the generally unwarranted deterministic power given to an autistic diagnosis, I often used an example taken from the schools: consider a student who has been diagnosed as dyslexic. One teacher might conclude that this student is incapable of learning to read, or nearly so. With a classroom of thirty-five students, that teacher will likely refrain from a full-out effort to teach that child to read, having assumed that it won't be possible to reach that goal. Consider another teacher in the same circumstance, who perceives the child behind the dyslexic symptoms, recognizes the child's strengths, such as tenacity in the face of challenges, and concludes that despite the diagnosis, this child just might be able to learn to read. Having seen the latent potential, that teacher will spare no effort to bring that child to literacy. Similarly, too often the diagnoses of autism, PDD or ASD run the risk of blinding practitioners to the realities of the child's full potential. Efforts to assist the child are then limited by the preconceptions regarding what is considered possible for a child diagnosed as autistic.

In the Feuerstein *dynamic* approach, the practitioner does not assume that diagnosing the child and understanding the child are necessarily equivalent. We might wish to assume that a formal diagnosis provides us with an understanding of a child, but this is not necessarily so, especially when we consider that the formal autism diagnostic criteria are so elastic and inclusive. Sometimes a conventional autism diagnosis provides merely a hypothesis.

This is not to imply that a diagnosis of autism, rooted in a stringent interpretation of Kanner's criteria—extreme emotional cutoffness, aloneness and obsessively perseverative behavior—is never applicable. Clearly, it can be. But a recurrent motif in this book is that the autism diagnosis is commonly applied too liberally. Working to uncover the strengths which may yet offset the child's difficulties, the dynamic practitioner is cautious in the application of this diagnosis. And when the diagnosis of autism, using stringent Kanner criteria, is found to be accurate, the dynamic practitioner proceeds in the same way as with children who present with mild to moderate autistiform symptoms: searching for and eliciting islets of normalcy on which to base further development.

In general, when working *dynamically*:

- The practitioner puts aside the pursuit of a diagnosis and focuses on understanding the child's situation.
- The dynamic assessor prioritizes a rich description of functioning, considers nuances of the child's difficulties, and seeks evidence of the child's strengths rather seeking to make a "closest fit" formal diagnosis.
- The practitioner in dynamic mode is aware that the autism diagnosis, rather than clarifying, often masks or obscures the child's difficulties—and strengths.
- Even in situations where a diagnosis of autism is appropriate, from the dynamic perspective, the assessor does not give the diagnosis the power to establish the child's developmental path.
- Generating evidence of positive potential, a profile of modifiability rather than a diagnosis, is the aim of a dynamic assessment, because we are working from the Feuerstein premise that autism is a state, not a trait, and as such is subject to modifiability.

Ben: A Dynamic Assessment and a Reconsidered Diagnosis

Before arriving at the Institute, Ben had already been through several conventional assessments which had utilized formal autism criteria. In all of these assessments, Ben had been diagnosed as PDD. Ben's parents had been overcome with distress following his diagnosis by autism specialists. Aware that the Feuerstein Institute staff worked from a different perspective regarding the potential modifiability of a child with developmental difficulties, they were anxious to hear our opinion: was Ben autistic or not? Before answering that question, I needed to explain to these parents the difficulties within conventional diagnostic criteria, and the working perspective of Feuerstein's dynamic approach. But first, I needed to observe Ben carefully, seeking islets of normalcy, getting a sense of his strengths as well as of his difficulties.

Mentally, I completely put the purported diagnosis of PDD aside and focused on Ben as an individual, here and now in my office. I did not want any preconceptions clouding my vision of who he really was. Ben's eye contact was steady. His eyes expressed trepidation, as might be expected from a child in a strange setting in the presence of a stranger. I made a mental note that trepidation denotes fear, and that fear denotes awareness of the world and of others. So his was not an instance of genuine autistic cutoffness.

Ben's body language, despite perhaps the tension of shyness, appeared normative. There were no perseverative (repetitive) behaviors such as hand-flapping, walking in circuits or any other behaviors that might be considered stereotypical in an autistic child. He was generally comfortable in his body.

Ben was quiet. He did not speak much. When he did, it appeared to be an emotional effort for him to trust himself. I began to imagine how in a conventional testing situation Ben might have acted withdrawn with a stranger who asked questions or who expected performance results. Withdrawn in apprehension and shyness, Ben's presentation might have looked far more serious than the one I observed. I hoped to draw him out further in this first session.

I invited Ben to sit at the table and join me in some "games" (play-based learning tasks). Although shy, Ben engaged well, if mostly quietly, during the interactional phase of this first session. He completed a number of kinder-garten level tasks, such as constructing puzzles, matching pictures, arranging pictures to form a story sequence and similar activities. He was able to remain reciprocal in a cautious but perceptible rhythm of give and take in communication with me, whether in his brief verbal responses or in his comprehending performance in the learning tasks. I was impressed by his quick aptitude with the repertoire of play-based learning activities. Despite his shyness, Ben appeared to enjoy what we were doing.

I mulled over my observations: shy; minimal but appropriate expressive language; capable of verbal reciprocity; no sense of emotional remoteness; normative body language with no perseverative or stereotypical movements; hesitant yet direct and emotionally laden eye contact. Though reticent and underconfident, Ben impressed as an emotionally present child who was not cut off. I soon ruled out autism. As for PDD, no longer in clinical use, this term was evidently used as an unfortunate and far too general catchall term for children who did not fit the formal criteria for autism in the *DSM-IV-TR*. I often felt that it offered neither clinical specificity nor a basis for formulating a differential diagnosis.

Having ruled out an autistic condition, I still felt at ease in not having an alternative diagnosis to pigeonhole his situation. I knew that I needed to share this attitude with his parents. Aware of the fact that Ben was lacking confidence and was far too reticent, I could see why he would be having difficulty when relating to peers in his kindergarten. He would need some good speech therapy to loosen the verbal channel as well as regular play dates at home with peers to build his social confidence. I hoped to continue following his progress until he was functioning in his educational setting commensurate with the potential I perceived.

Ben's parents would also require our help. First of all, they needed to understand that Ben's situation was not one of autism or its near synonym at the time, PDD. They would then need recommendations attuned to my perception of Ben's abilities. I spent the rest of the session explaining to Ben's parents how the overly elastic criteria for PDD had resulted in his misdiagnosis. I acknowledged his shy and quiet demeanor, but I highlighted his involved, engaged functioning on some basic learning tasks as a key strength. I recommended that Ben continue to be integrated in his regular kindergarten and that he not be transferred to a special kindergarten among communication-impaired youngsters as other experts had strongly recommended.

Ben's parents, so shaken by the conventional diagnosis they had received from other settings, yearned to accept my interpretation of their child's difficulties, needs and strengths. But emotionally they could not completely do so. The power of a diagnosis of autism is very great in the minds of many.

There are times when it is important to put one's ego aside. This was one of them. I needed help to reach these parents. Professor Feuerstein possessed an indefatigable commitment to promoting his methods of learning and treatment which were based on the intrinsic capacity of the human being for modifiability. He shared this wisdom generously not only with his staff but also with the many parents and children who frequented the Institute. I had often picked up the phone in the middle of an assessment session to ask whether he might be available to see a child and to contribute his insights from his wealth of knowledge and experience. It was clear that my interpretation of Ben's situation would not be enough to move his parents from a place of deep doubt about the essential abilities of their son, given the pall of the formal diagnosis. I phoned the Professor's direct line and briefly explained the situation. He agreed to see Ben immediately.

As he observed Ben in his office, the Professor concluded as well: Ben should not be considered autistic or PDD, and it was imperative that he continue in his regular kindergarten. The combined impact of Feuerstein's authoritative personality, his deep compassion, the depth and breadth of his clinical wisdom and the benefit of his over fifty years' experience helped the parents embrace what would ultimately prove to be for them and for Ben a life-saving paradigm shift.

Following their encounter with the Professor, the parents agreed to bring Ben for periodic follow-up sessions at the Institute. Of critical importance, they decided to accept our recommendations to maintain Ben in his regular kindergarten. Despite lurking doubts, they were open to our interpretation of their son's challenges that did not involve the formal categorization of his presentation into pathology. They were responsive to a perspective that discerned evident strengths and intuited latent abilities, and which gave greater credence to these strengths and abilities than to their child's difficulties.

Differing Assumptions, Expectations and Prognoses

Over the years, in reviewing the referral information of hundreds of children, I found that the *conventional* assumptions, expectations and prognoses related to autism, as reflected in practitioners' reports, were typified by:

- A doubtful attitude toward the child's potential for developmental change.
- Assumed poor prognoses for children with autistiform symptoms which in turn influenced the treatment and placement recommendations.
- Generally pessimistic assumptions regarding the condition of autism as not significantly changeable: "This child does not/cannot understand." "She will never talk normally." "Hand-flapping is part of who he is."
- A professional stance mindful of a doctor's relaying news of a "terminal" condition.

Too often an autistic condition appeared to be considered in conventional circles as essentially incurable. One might be able to change certain skill levels, but according to the conventional way of thinking about autism, changing the essential nature and personality of the child, his or her way of being in the world, does not really change. "Your child will always be autistic" parents are told, or have read on the internet. From our experience of many years, and as the cases in this book illustrate, this is not necessarily true!

During intake sessions, I have met so many parents who wept as they coped with the angst of a report they had received elsewhere "confirming" an autistic diagnosis. Many had arrived at their own negative prognostic thoughts: "He is mentally impaired." "They said that my child was born like this, and that she will always be autistic. But I remember how lively she was at her birthday party last year." "He will never be completely independent." And in line with this pessimistic stance, these parents had received negative and discouraging advice and recommendations.

One of the most blatant examples of poor advice based on a practitioner's pessimistic assumptions still echoes loudly in my memory. The mother of a child diagnosed elsewhere as autistic wept as she told my colleague that in the summary meeting following her son's conventional assessment and diagnosis, she had been advised: "Don't bother talking to your child. He doesn't understand language. He's autistic. It's like talking to the wall." Incidentally, my speech therapist colleague counseled her to do precisely the opposite: "Your child's condition can be improved. He must hear your voice. Speak to your child!"

The *dynamic approach* offers a positive perspective, useful strategies and a sense of hope with even the more challenging presentations:

- The dynamic practitioner works from the assumption that the condition of the child, like any human being, is inherently modifiable.
- The prognosis then becomes much more positive and optimistic. When one expects and seeks positive change, it is more likely to occur.
- Neither the prognosis nor expectations are limited to the pessimistic preconceptions that often attach to the term "autistic."
- Because the work in the Feuerstein paradigm is based on the concept that autism is a condition, a modifiable state and not an unchangeable trait,[5] we anticipate the capacity for modifiability in a child beyond the severity of the presenting symptoms or the given diagnosis.

Regarding autism as a trait versus a state, Feuerstein explained that when you have a cold, for example, you are in a condition—a state—of having a cold. You do not remain in that state forever. Having a cold is not who you are. The cold can get better. It is the quality and quantity of the mediation, that energetic, intentional involvement with the child, which has the potential to change what appeared at first to be an ingrained trait to a modifiable state.

This is not naïve optimism coupled with a wait-and-see attitude. In the dynamic paradigm, optimism goes hand in hand with the hard work of seeking and eliciting islets of normalcy, guided by a vision of the positive potential of the child behind the symptoms. It is the evidence of strengths, the islets of normalcy, that ultimately give the practitioner working dynamically the platform on which to base more promising prognoses and recommendations attuned to individual needs and strengths. Because in-session we have observed and/or created evidence of the child's modifiability, we can confidently anticipate further positive change.

This prompts a few questions. Does this mean that every child with an accurate autism diagnosis, as per a strict interpretation of Kanner's criteria, can be brought to normative functioning and face a normative future? No, there are situations which are stubborn, complex, compounded by physiological limitations, and/or compromised by limited treatment options. But the practitioner working from a dynamic perspective will invest proportionally much more energy to elicit strengths when a child's presentation is challenging to try to improve that presentation.

Does this mean that every child diagnosed as autistic is not autistic? No. There are children who are genuinely autistic, again, using a strict interpretation of Kanner's criteria. But in my twenty-five years at the Institute, I encountered far fewer genuinely autistic children than the current statistics for the "autism epidemic" reflect.[6,7]

Does this mean that every child diagnosed as autistic and who receives proper treatment can become absolutely normal? No. But it does mean that meaningful change and improvement are possible, even in the key areas of autism, namely, verbal communication, social cutoffness and perseverative behaviors. It can mean that severe symptoms can become less so, moderate or mild. It can also mean that a child who is considered "somewhat" autistic can entirely shed the shadow and impact of what appeared at first to be a relevant ASD diagnosis.

Related to this discussion of expectations and assumptions is a term I frequently encountered in referral material, the notion of "high functioning autism," which I would like to put briefly under the microscope. In my work, I sensed that the shadow of negative assumptions, lowered expectations and compromised prognoses associated with lower functioning autistic children had attached to these higher functioning children, whose strengths and overall developmental health were often impressive. Some of the children diagnosed as "autistic, high functioning" did exhibit some peculiarities of behavior, though not necessarily with an autistic nuance; that is, they were not verbally uncommunicative, emotionally cut off or perseverative. In many cases, the children presented normatively. They were highly expressive verbally and evidenced appropriate social skills. In fact, some of these "high functioning autistic" children were talented and unique personalities. Some were even gifted. Others perhaps exhibited slight idiosyncrasies of personality (for example, the child prefers stamp collecting to playing hide-and-seek or talks only about rocket ships) but they did not meet Kanner's criteria for a genuine autistic condition. Nevertheless, they were still bearing the label "high functioning autism" with all the connotations of impairment that the term elicits in the minds of many parents and teachers. And for some children, the diagnosis of "high functioning autism" seemed to trail them in the educational system like a shadow long after they had jettisoned any idiosyncratic developmental features.

It is unfortunate that many assessing practitioners emphasize a child's unusual behaviors and categorize these "high functioning" and presumably autistic children on the "impaired" side of the equation, rather than considering the child's strengths, and describing a child, for example, as "a talented child, with some unique interests, who would benefit from therapeutic gymnastics in order to give him opportunities for active, energetic peer contacts." What is at work here psychologically? My hunch is that the answer is in no small part the preconceptions, expectations and self-fulfilling prophecies deriving from the power of a diagnosis.

When we internalize the imperative of the human capacity for modifiability, and when we then seek the child's islets of normalcy, the shadows and preconceptions of the autism diagnosis melt away and make room for our active, optimistic engagement with the energies of the child. It is one of the mantras of this book that it will not be the diagnosis that will determine the child's progress. It will be the child's own strengths and energies, coupled with our objective to work beyond conventional expectations and assumptions in order to reach the child behind the symptoms.

Ben: Alternative Assumptions, Expectations and Prognoses

Ben's parents entered the Institute struggling with a set of assumptions and expectations which were embedded in a shadowy prognosis. They left the Institute that first day hopeful yet still struggling, as they sought to embrace a different perspective of their child's difficulties. The Professor and I had perceived Ben's latent strengths, those islets of normalcy—his ability to engage, his capacity for reciprocity, his enjoyment of learning tasks—in the sea of his weaknesses, namely, shyness, low confidence and reticent verbalization, that had translated into poor social communication skills. We believed that Ben's expressive language and his social skills would ultimately flourish with added speech therapy and play dates, along with his continued educational integration, with all the stimulation and challenges that offered. Belief in Ben, of itself, would not have been enough, as belief might only be a function of wishful thinking. But in the dynamic assessment process just begun, we had carefully observed and interacted with Ben, all the while weighing his subtle, latent strengths against his difficulties. Only after we had observed Ben's strengths and highlighted their relative predominance in his profile were we in a position to envision a positive prognosis for Ben.

Differing Outlooks on Causality (Etiology)

Simply put, etiology means the root cause of a disease or condition. What causes autism? This question itself is problematic since the criteria which clinically define autism have expanded enormously from their more restricted beginnings in 1943. A researcher probing genetic or physiological correlates of autism using an "autistic population" which has been selected according to the hyper-elastic and widely inclusive formal diagnostic criteria would be hard-pressed to know whether his or her research subjects are in fact truly autistic, or rather are suffering from a broad range of other social communication difficulties. Nevertheless, scientists are hard at work in the fields of biology, biochemistry, neurology and genetics in an effort to identify the specific biological causes of autism.[8,9]

The *conventional* assumption is that there must be a specific gene, brain peculiarity or biochemical trigger that causes autism. That assumption appears to rest on a conceptualization of autism as an "it," a trait which must be innate, or at least in some way biologically determined. According to this worldview, although cosmetic changes might be made to a child's presentation, essentially the child is born with such-and-such a gene, brain structure or biochemical configuration and therefore will remain irrevocably autistic.

What is the response to such research findings by practitioners working in the *dynamic* paradigm? Years ago, when explaining to a French reporter the impact of biological givens from his dynamic perspective, Feuerstein meaningfully quipped: "I will never give the chromosome the last word."[10] This simplistic sounding sentence is actually quite profound. Feuerstein never denied the influence of genetic material or physiological facts on the human being. Rather, he maintained that the environment, specifically the intentional human input, has the power to influence and even overcome many of the effects of heredity. The active, focused mediational involvement of the parent, teacher or practitioner has the power to profoundly affect the cognitive and general developmental potential of the individual, beyond the impact of biological givens.

Does this mean that someone with Down syndrome will then shed the syndrome if he or she receives the proper interventions? No, but it does mean that energetic and optimistic interventions, sensitive to the latent potential of an individual, can elicit a level of functioning much higher than the physiological givens suggest. Thus, at the Institute, my colleagues and I witnessed many Down syndrome children learning to read and then integrating in typical elementary schools; brain-injured soldiers recovering unexpectedly large capacities for thinking and functioning given the extent of their injuries; children with congenital deficits achieving cognitively at a level far beyond the textbook expectations of their deficits; and children who had been diagnosed as "autistic spectrum" going on to lead normal or near normal childhoods.

Research teams are hard at work to discover definitive genetic, biochemical and other causes of autism. Will the findings prove that these factors must establish the child's future? Even if a particular gene or biochemical marker is "proven" to cause autism, from the Feuerstein perspective, that gene or marker will only be considered a potential influence on the child's functioning but not a determinant of the child's identity, abilities or destiny.

Many years ago my colleagues and I had the privilege of attending several of the remarkable conferences on autism organized in conjunction with ICDL by the originators of DIR, Stanley Greenspan and Serena Wieder. At one conference there were twelve hundred participants, including parents of autistic children and practitioners from many fields, who came to listen to cutting-edge presentations by research scientists, doctors, therapists and parents—all focused on the subject of autism.

One presentation was particularly memorable—that of a physician who had been researching the physiological correlates of autism for years, and who presented impressive research data on the differing biochemical and brain variations of autistic versus non-autistic children. At the end of his fascinating presentation, I approached him with a question: "Are the differences in brain and biological markers the cause of autism? Or are they the physiological results of chronically impaired developmental functioning, common to children considered autistic? Are we dealing with biochemical/brain correlates which are a *cause* or an *effect* of autism?" Pleased with the question, he responded, "That is an important question, one which I wish I could answer." From a dynamic perspective, we treat the scientific findings of physiological correlates of autism with respect, as noteworthy, suspected influences of an autistic condition, but not as inevitable determinants of the child's future functioning.

Ben: Predetermined or Promising?

Ben's referral information and his parents' own verbal reports to us did not include any reference to suspected genetic, neurological or physiological complications in Ben's background. Had I noticed "soft signs" of such complications, such as Ben's blanking out in neurologically rooted absences, seriously delayed motor milestones, dysmorphia (pronounced asymmetry) in his facial features, or other unusual physiological signs, I would have been quick to recommend to his parents a consultation with a relevant medical specialist to clarify Ben's physical situation and/or to rule out certain conditions. At the same time, had that been the case, I would have been equally quick to educate the parents in the dynamic way of looking at such influences: namely, that a particular syndrome or neurological condition might influence the child's development but need not limit the child's potential. In our work, the chromosome did not get the last word.

With Ben's normative medical profile, his situation clearly had emotional roots (his shyness, underconfidence and reticence) rather than genetic or other physiological roots. Even with this understanding there was a sense of mystery. His parents were impressive in the degree of love, understanding and devotion to him that they communicated. There was no history of trauma, either physical or emotional. The roots of Ben's verbal reticence and social weaknesses were not clear. What was clear in that initial observation and interaction with him, and in successive sessions with him in the year following, was that Ben was capable of strengthening his fragile but nevertheless normative abilities.

Differing Modes of Intervention

It is beyond the scope of this book to provide an overview of the various extant methods of working with children thought to be autistic. In this section, I wish simply to distinguish between two general outlooks on their treatment: skill-based training models versus models based on reciprocity which search for an overall shift in the child's propensity to communicate and function. *Skill-training methods* would seem to be rooted in a perspective which views autism as an innate trait, unchangeable in its essence. Perhaps that is why these methods focus primarily on skill development, such as learning to use picture symbols, learning to begin and complete a given task, learning to say "good morning" to the teacher.

At a workshop years ago, Serena Wieder cautioned against the reduction of therapeutic goals to what she called "splinter skills,"[11] such as, "the child will learn to use the pronoun 'I'" or "the child will maintain eye contact for ten seconds" or "the child will accept sitting beside the teacher." While these aspects may be important to a child's functioning, DIR considers the development of the whole child—relationship, feelings, personality and skills as well—although the latter are always sought within the context of the whole person and the dynamics of a real, vibrant interpersonal relationship replete with circles of communication.

The *dynamic* Feuerstein method similarly prioritizes the *process* of learning and reciprocal communication over the *products* of learning, such as IQ scores or particular skill acquisition. This approach encourages the practitioner to aim for deeper and more substantive changes in the child's overall propensity to communicate and function. My colleagues and I would not select reading per se as a goal, but reading as an expression of the child's overall ability to think and process. We would not target "a vocabulary of ten words" as a goal, but rather work energetically to mediate a greater openness in the child to verbal communication. We would not mechanically try to induce more sustained eye contact, but rather work with humor, warmth and playfulness to elicit the desire in the child for closer contact and reciprocity.

It is the strong bias of this book that methods which prize the growth of personhood, personality and relationship are preferable to methods which target skill acquisition in children with autistiform features. Often skill acquisition methods rely on training through repetition. Many behavioral practitioners now incorporate the warmth of an interpersonal relationship into their skill training protocols with children. This is a noteworthy shift in a developmentally sound direction.

Differing Advice and Recommendations to Parents

My observations about the types of recommendations commonly given to parents from a *conventional* perspective are based on my long-term interface with the Israeli educational system while working for twenty-five years at an institute which embraced an alternative mode of psychology and human development. Because the following observations pertain to the predominant Israeli experience, they may not apply to all countries and cultures.

In Israel, referral or assessment reports from practitioners working from a *conventional* perspective invariably recommended speech and occupational therapy for the child with autistiform symptoms, and guidance sessions to help the parents with their child's suspected autism. Most pertinently, these reports routinely recommended the child's placement within a special school or class for autistic children.

Within the Israeli educational system, there are legions of devoted educators and therapists at all levels of practice and administration. However, the current policy of the system as a whole is to create special classes for children with special needs. Although educational integration is legally available in Israel, it is weakly supported within the national budget. Yet even given these fiscal constraints, there exist talented teachers who are willing to include a child with special needs in their regular classes. There are open-minded principals and superintendents of regular schools who support such integration. There are a modest number of fully integrated settings, particularly kindergartens, some of which are private. But in general, the current prevalent expectation in Israel is that a child with special needs will be placed in a smaller special classroom, among peers with similar special needs according to diagnostic category, such as learning disabled, cognitively impaired, autistic, and so on. Although special settings are enriched by having onsite therapists, lacking in our estimation is the critical element of typical peers who can serve as role models for the challenged child's imitation of normative speech, communication, cognition, play and socialization.

From a *dynamic perspective*, my colleagues and I attempted to provide parents with a comprehensive action plan, with practical, individually attuned recommendations, ideas and strategies for helping their child, which covered an extensive range of developmental areas: verbal and nonverbal communication; interactive play development; socialization readiness; and underlying health issues, such as vision or hearing acuity, or food sensitivities. Although referrals for more intensive DIR intervention and basic interventions such as speech and occupational therapy were often recommended, it was particularly important for us to empower the parents and to provide them with specific mediational techniques which they could incorporate and use with their child within their daily routine. We attempted to generate recommendations attuned to the specific needs, personality and strengths of each individual child and of the parents. In successive follow-up sessions, our recommendations and pointers to parents were revised in accordance with the rate and extent of the child's developmental progress.

The need for parents to internalize and utilize Feuerstein's concept of verbal soliloquy was a key recommendation. I encouraged parents simply to "talk to your child." At the same time, I suggested to skeptical, worried parents to simply "observe" the effect of this talking to their child amply and richly over the course of the next several weeks—without embracing huge expectations, in order to protect parents from any initial disappointment. Often this mini-intervention at home on the part of the parent led to encouraging changes in the child: better eye contact, more babbling, verbal utterances, and so on. Feeling encouraged, parents were then more likely to accept advice from our perspective emphasizing potential and modifiability.

However, our linchpin recommendation for the educational placement of a child with autistiform symptoms was usually that of integration (inclusion). In practice, what this meant was that at the Institute my colleagues and I often recommended educational integration to parents who were interfacing with a system which was geared to provide homogeneously organized special needs classes.

We, the Institute staff, were always swimming upstream against the prevalent current. But we were committed to our direction. Other professionals who had previously assessed the child in conventional fashion had as a matter of course strongly recommended special education for the child. But having glimpsed the child behind the symptoms and having observed meaningful examples of the child's potential for change, in the majority of cases, though not all, we recommended educational integration, often with the addition of varying levels of in-class or at-home supports for the child, such as an integration aide or additional therapies.

From the Feuerstein perspective, a regular classroom or social setting becomes a "modifying environment," with the energy, interaction, challenges and higher expectations of a normative group pulling the child with developmental challenges to a higher level of functioning.[12] Our follow-up services to parents included as much support for the child's educational integration as possible, in the form of our dialoguing with a child's regular classroom teacher advising the integration aide, meeting with school staff and attending pivotal educational placement meetings.

By shifting one's paradigmatic perspective and the methods of working that result from that shift, no one can promise parents that their child with autistic features will achieve normal or near normal functioning. However, if in the course of the dynamic assessment sessions my colleagues and I have been able to demonstrate to the parents that their child possesses previously overlooked islets of normalcy, and in these sessions we have observed evidence of modifiability, then we will work to encourage parents to try to make that paradigm shift so that we can realize the maximum possible potential.

Ben: Method of Working, Our Recommendations —And the Results

Ben clearly required some support to enhance his evident though fragile normative social communication abilities, but he was not in need of skill-based behavioral strategies. His personality and confidence needed to be strengthened in a normative, relational context. Contrary to the recommendations embedded in the reports of previous specialists, I did not recommend for Ben a slew of therapies, such as speech therapy, occupational therapy, therapeutic horseback riding and so on. Certainly, these types of therapies can be critically important in the lives of many children. But for Ben it did not appear advisable to develop his language and social skills in technical fashion. Rather, these needed to be developed within a rich, even if challenging, social context—that of educational integration.

Had Ben's parents adopted the recommendations of the previous specialists and enrolled him in a small class composed entirely of children with communication impairments or autistiform features, Ben would have received frequent speech therapy there. However, he would have been placed among other communication-challenged children. He would have lacked a rich and stimulating social milieu in which to incubate and integrate the skills he was being taught. Although socialization with peers did not come easily for Ben, I concluded that he would benefit from the ongoing challenge and enrichment which his current normative peer setting offered. Such a setting would challenge him but it would also stretch him and impel him to change. It seemed reasonable to believe that Ben could succeed in his typical setting without an integration aide, and he did.

I offered his parents other recommendations, those that stressed the dynamic way of nurturing Ben's latent strengths. I urged them to step outside the shadow of the doubts that the formal PDD diagnosis had cast and to relate to their son with all the naturalness and warmth they showed their other children. So often I have seen parents of children who have been given a formal diagnosis with an autistic nuance unconsciously pull back emotionally from their child. Parents sometimes then doubt their own natural abilities for warmth and love, fearing that they have to do everything "just right" in order to relate to their child in a matter compatible with a given diagnosis.[13]

Our message to Ben's parents was to trust their feelings and their well-honed parenting instincts. I reminded them of the importance of speaking to him amply, using a rich vocabulary and modeling full normative language. I strongly recommended that Ben have play dates at home, preferably twice a week, with one or two of the children from his kindergarten. Back in his kindergarten, he would then find faces familiar to him from home and encounter children with whom he already shared a basis of play interaction.

Ben: Epilogue

I continued to follow Ben's progress with follow-up observation and interactional sessions for about a year and a half. During that time, Ben required an additional year in a regular kindergarten to consolidate the gains he had made during the year he first arrived at the Institute. Later, his first grade experience proved difficult. His weaknesses in self-confidence, verbal expression and social connections haunted him. Fortunately, his teacher was open to phone dialogue and consultation with us, and I was able to provide her not only with encouragement about Ben's abilities but also about her own abilities to support Ben. Ben's parents had decided not to disclose to his new school that Ben had once been misdiagnosed as PDD. All too often, the power of a diagnosis impacts negatively on the natural abilities and instincts of good educators. As it turned out, Ben's first grade teacher considered him a typical, if underconfident, child. By the end of first grade, Ben had strengthened and improved. Although not at the top of his class, he was participating in activities, learning well and sustaining appropriate contact with peers. Shortly afterward, Ben's parents stopped bringing him to the Institute, and their phone updates to us tapered off as well.

Years passed. Roughly ten years later, while culling old files, I came across Ben's name and his parents' phone number. I could not resist phoning them to hear how Ben's life had evolved. The news was very good. Ben was now an outstanding high school student, well-liked by his peers. His parents were thankful for the call. They were effusive in their thanks to the Professor and me for being the only ones from among the many professionals who had seen Ben to have identified the misdiagnosis and to have urged them to keep their son in the regular educational system. They were the proud and happy parents of a teen whose early childhood developmental challenges had faded and then disappeared as his latent abilities emerged.

The happy ending of Ben's story turned out to be even happier. Many years later, I heard my name being called as I was pulling my luggage off the carousel at airport arrivals, "Doctor Shoshana!" It was Ben's parents. They were beaming at the opportunity to once again express their deepest appreciation that we had perceived the inaccuracy of Ben's formal autism diagnosis and that we had supported them in making a paradigm shift in their perception of and treatment decisions for their son. They wanted to show me some photos. Ben's mother pulled out her cellphone. The happy faces of Ben and his wife, holding their newborn son, smiled back at me. For Ben, the paradigm shift had indeed been life-saving.

Notes

1 Most commonly these are the Autism Behavior Checklist (ABC), the Childhood Autism Rating Scale (CARS) and the Checklist for Autism in Toddlers (M-CHAT), as referred to in earlier chapters.
2 Catherine Lord et al., *Autism Diagnostic Observation Schedule, ADOS-2* (Torrance, CA: Western Psychological Services, 2012).
3 Ibid., 119.
4 Mandia Mentis, Marilyn J. Dunn-Bernstein, and Martene Mentis, *Mediated Learning: Teaching, Tasks, and Tools to Unlock Cognitive Potential* (Thousand Oaks, CA: Corwin, 2008).
5 Rafael S. Feuerstein, ed., *Feuerstein on Autism* (Jerusalem: Feuerstein Institute, 2019).
6 Matthew J. Maenner et al., "Prevalence of Autism Spectrum Disorder among Children Aged 8 Years—Autism and Developmental Disabilities Monitoring Network, 11 Sites, United States, 2016," *MMWR Surveillance Summaries* 69, no. SS-4 (2020): 1–12.
7 Steve Silberman, *NeuroTribes: The Legacy of Autism and the Future of Neurodiversity* (New York: Penguin Random House, 2015).
8 James Lyons-Weiler, *The Environmental and Genetic Causes of Autism* (New York: Skyhorse, 2016).
9 Salvatore A. Currenti, "Understanding and Determining the Etiology of Autism," *Cell and Molecular Neurobiology*, no. 30 (2010): 161-71. Consideration of the numerous findings of autism-related research is beyond the scope of this book, whose focus is to document children's progress within a population whose ability to progress significantly is often doubted. The sources in notes 8 and 9 are included as representative of such research.
10 Reuven Feuerstein and Antoine Spire, *La Pedagogie a Visage Humain* (Paris: La Bord de L'Eau, 2006).
11 Serena Wieder, personal communication to author (2020). This term was used by Dr. Wieder at a professional training seminar whose original date proved untraceable.
12 Reuven Feuerstein, "Shaping Modifying Environments Through Inclusion," *Transylvanian Journal of Psychology*, Special Issue No. 2 (2007): 9–23.

13 The parents of Jack (Chapter 1) are a classic example of this occurrence. Their relationship with Jack suffered a huge setback after Jack received an autism-related diagnosis. Before the conventional assessment, they delighted in him. After the diagnosis, they pulled back from him emotionally, seriously doubting the abilities of their son, and their own ability to parent him. It took them several years to recover their own confidence and their delight in him.

References

Currenti, Salvatore A. "Understanding and Determining the Etiology of Autism." *Cell and Molecular Neurobiology* 30 (2010): 161–71.

Feuerstein, Rafael S., ed., *Feuerstein on Autism.* Jerusalem: Feuerstein Institute, 2019.

Feuerstein, Reuven. "Shaping Modifying Environments through Inclusion." *Transylvanian Journal of Psychology*, Special Issue No. 2 (2007): 9–23.

Feuerstein, Reuven and Antoine Spire. *La Pedagogie a Visage Humain.* Paris: La Bord de L'Eau, 2006.

Lord, Catherine, Michael Rutter, Pamela C. Dilavore, Susan Risi, Katherine Gotham, and Somer L. Bishop. *Autism Diagnostic Observation Schedule, ADOS-2.* Torrance, CA: Western Psychological Services, 2012.

Lyons-Weiler, James. *The Environmental and Genetic Causes of Autism.* New York: Skyhorse, 2016.

Maenner, Matthew J., Kelly A. Shaw, Jon Baio, Anita Washington, Mary Patrick, Monica DiRienzo, Deborah L. Christensen et al. "Prevalence of Autism Spectrum Disorder Among Children Aged 8 Years—Autism and Developmental Disabilities Monitoring Network, 11 Sites, United States, 2016." *MMWR Surveillance Summaries* 69, no. 4 (2020): 1–12.

Mentis, Mandia, Marilyn J. Dunn-Bernstein, and Martene Mentis. *Mediated Learning: Teaching, Tasks, and Tools to Unlock Cognitive Potential.* Thousand Oaks, CA: Corwin, 2008.

Silberman, Steve. *NeuroTribes: The Legacy of Autism and the Future of Neurodiversity.* New York: Penguin Random House, 2015.

16 Concluding Reflections

In the Introduction, I likened my generation-long career to working in the trenches. Trenches evoke images of dark, muddy murkiness and back-breaking labor. Yet in the trenches of the nitty-gritty challenges of daily work, playfully wooing children with autistic features upward toward improved functioning and their parents toward strengthened interactions with the children, there was light in the form of inspiration—from the theoretical outlook, methods and insights of Feuerstein, into which I opted to interweave the play-based developmental strategies of Greenspan and Wieder. In relaying the stories of the children in this casebook, I have drawn from the assessment and treatment dramas that unfolded within the confines of my office. But there were also gifted colleagues, and together we worked with hundreds of other children who presented with autistiform symptoms. So there was not only the light of inspiration but also the delight and the satisfaction we shared in seeing the lives of so many children with developmental challenges change for the better.

Jack, Sasha, Annie, Davie, Joe, Mikey, Max and Josh. Ernie, Sammy, Ben, Amy, Gordie and Leo. Each child is a world unto him- or herself, and each case story has something unique to teach us. Retrospectively considering these children's stories and reviewing the trajectories of their progress, it is noteworthy that some of these children were seen for barely a few assessment sessions and perhaps intermittently for a few more follow-up sessions. Ordinarily, the mandate of the Feuerstein Institute is to offer a generous series of assessment sessions and then long-term developmental follow-up. My colleagues and I usually saw young children many times over a course of a year or two at least, with occasional follow-ups in later childhood and beyond not uncommon. Yet as these case stories illustrate, sometimes even within a single assessment session there was movement. Something dislodged. Something happened that shifted the developmental trajectory away from the presenting difficulties and pathology, and *toward* normative functioning, even if the first islet of normalcy noticed or elicited was microscopically small and fleetingly brief. And something shifted within the parents as well.

Why? What worked? What accounted for the earlier modest and, later, often dramatic changes? What confluence of factors conspired to help these autistiform but, as it emerged in most cases, not autistic children begin to shed worrisome symptoms and become more attuned, communicative and functional? What was happening in these early sessions that enabled and encouraged the parents to pursue the therapies, interventions and educational settings, usually inclusive, that would help create a more normative profile for their child in the years to come? What did we do that helped?

The short answer to these questions, I believe, lies in the fact that we exposed the parents to a different way of perceiving their child, through the lens of strength and promise rather than through the lens of pathology. The composite answers to these questions have been considered throughout this book, embedded in each child's tale. However, in this concluding chapter I attempt to summarize, reflect on and further develop the answers to these questions as they pertain in interdependent fashion to parents, practitioners and the children. In the reflections following, the admixture of theoretical versus practical aspects varies, with a strong inclination toward the practical, to help ease parents and practitioners toward the recommended paradigm shift that this casebook encourages.

The Impact on Parents of a Child's Autism Diagnosis

In the most practical terms, in anticipation of meeting parents arriving with their child for the first time, I learned that I needed to have at the ready a pile of tissues for parents' tears. Receiving an autism-related diagnosis, whether the now obsolete AD, Asperger's and PDD, or the current ASD, was usually a blow to the parents I saw that ranged from difficult to devastating. Raising a child with any type of special needs can be challenging and distressing for parents. However, while working for many years with children who presented with a wide range of developmental difficulties, I observed that the various diagnoses related to autism seemed to carry an extra heavy emotional valence for parents. I met so many parents whose thoughts about their child's AD or ASD diagnosis had revved into a paralyzing combination of panic and fear: "My child is unreachable." "My child has no future." "My child will not be independent, marry or have a normal life." Such thoughts, to varying degrees, were clearly weighing on the parents of Jack, Sasha, Annie, Davie, Joe, Mikey, Max and Josh. Usually my first task in helping the child was to help the parents counter the impact of these troubling thoughts, which are not at all necessarily true!

Serena Wieder, co-developer of DIRFloortime, has spoken of some parents occasionally going into a period of confusion or grief after receiving an autism diagnosis of their child.[1] If a child is diagnosed at the age of two and if, to suggest an arbitrary example, it takes a parent two years to recover from attendant feelings that might range from discouragement to hopelessness and then to galvanize their energy into a proactive program to help their child, two crucial years of child development have gone by, during which time so much could have been done to improve the child's developmental prognosis and during which time the child, above all, needed the parents' energy and positive emotional presence. And what if the autism diagnosis had been applied too liberally or was simply incorrect?

Parents are not at fault here. My experience taught that the highly generalized, highly elastic formal criteria for autism have created a situation in which too many children who present with an enormous range of developmental and communication difficulties are misdiagnosed as autistic. This is not to say that genuine autism, rooted in a stringent interpretation of Kanner's original and succinct formulation of this condition, with two primary criteria of emotional cutoffness and obsessive perseveration, does not exist. It does. However, clinical experience in encountering many children with social communication impairments almost daily for nearly twenty-five years led me to estimate that as many as ninety percent of the children with autistiform symptoms whom I saw had elsewhere been misdiagnosed as autistic using formal criteria or symptom checklists. I wanted parents to understand how a misdiagnosis of autism can occur so frequently, in order to give them the perspective to free themselves, at least in part, from the discouragement a formal autism diagnosis often conveys.

Even the accurate diagnosis of a genuinely autistic condition need not have the tragic implications for a child's future, as some parents fear; similarly with children whose autistiform symptoms appear together (comorbidly) with genetic or neurological conditions. While the prognoses may be more guarded in these situations, and the necessary treatment more intensive, even in such situations, my experience taught, there is much that can be done to help a child. The frequent, in fact rampant, misdiagnosis and overuse of the term autism with children who present with a vast range of developmental/communication/emotional delays, weaknesses and deficits does have a potentially tragic aspect as it relates to clinical practice, in my opinion.

The weighty and often pessimistic assumptions and presumptions that usually attach to the term "autistic" or the current "autistic spectrum" or sometimes even just "spectrum" often impact negatively on parents. The cart then pulls the horse. That is, misconceptions about the child who presents with only mild autistiform symptoms, as being necessarily unreachable or "incurable"—assumptions frequently associated with children with extremely challenging autistiform presentations—then attach to the diagnosis of the significantly less-impaired child. It is even possible that the frustrations and sense of pessimism experienced by some clinicians who have worked with children who present with severe, stubborn autistiform symptoms are then ascribed to children who present with mild to moderate symptoms. Often, rather than the prioritization of creative and in-depth clinical understanding of the child's comprehensive developmental situation, and the search for the child's strengths, the diagnosis then becomes the overarching influence for treatment intervention and educational placement. The diagnosis, sometimes the misdiagnosis, rather than the child's own strengths and ability to grow and change, essentially operates as a definition of who the child is and serves as a major determinant of the child's future.

Throughout my career, it was not uncommon to encounter children for whom the autism diagnosis appeared to have sealed their fate. The diagnosis rather than the child's latent and incipient strengths were influencing the treatment and placement goals. This was a phenomenon which deeply concerned Reuven Feuerstein, who believed that "traditional diagnoses emanating from the psychiatric and educational communities served to close off the potential of [a clinician's] response to [children's] optimistic potentials and, through their labels, imprison people in underperforming and unpotentialized lives."[2]

The reader might ask: Isn't this how it should be? Isn't it the diagnosis that we should be seeking? Doesn't a diagnosis name and therefore clarify my child's situation? Why shouldn't the diagnosis of autism signal to me as a parent that my child needs all of the interventions, treatments and services usually recommended for autistic spectrum children? This might be so if a developmental diagnosis related to autism offered the same degree of scientific clarity as with the diagnosis of physical illness. But as this book has striven to illustrate, this is not necessarily so.

Generally, we can trust that the results of medical tests will lead to a clear diagnosis. The doctor will use this diagnosis to determine the intervention. This may be true enough, though not infallibly so, in the field of medicine, where the advances of biochemistry and medical technology provide a high degree of analytical resolution. However, the tools of diagnosis regarding the developmental condition called "autism" are far less specific and exact than the tools of medicine, despite the repeated attempts to refine and recategorize the formal diagnostic symptoms. And that is why one of my first goals in an initial meeting with the parents of a child who had received an autism-related diagnosis was to help them understand the generalizations embedded in the recent versions of the formal diagnostic autism criteria.

Supporting the Parents: From Diagnosis, to Islets, to Action

Supporting the parents toward adopting an alternative way of looking at autism and a more dynamic, positive way of working with the child was crucial in order to create developmental momentum. There were three main components: educating parents about the weaknesses inherent in the formal autism diagnostic criteria and about the limitations of a diagnosis; helping parents to identify and to elicit islets of normalcy; and providing parents with strategic advice and recommendations that were feasible for them to carry out.

Along the lines of the discussion in Chapter 13, I often engaged parents in a close reading of the formal autism diagnostic criteria, discussing with them some of the embedded imprecision and overgeneralization. The aim was not to disparage the formal criteria but to educate parents in order to empower and strengthen them, to help them understand the fragility of a diagnosis that rests on highly flexible criteria.

Even when my observations of a severely cut off, noncommunicative, perseverative child—using a stringent interpretation of Kanner's criteria—indicated that the child was genuinely autistic (like Leo, Chapter 12), I reminded parents of a key Feuerstein tenet, that autism is a state—amenable to change and modifiability—not an indelibly etched trait. If a parent held that an autism diagnosis was the summation of their child, we ran the risk of hitting the glass ceiling of preconceptions, such as "my child will never ...," which are not necessarily true.

Does that mean that all autistic children can shed all traces of their difficulties and proceed to lead normal, independent lives? It does not. However, if in the course of seeking islets of normalcy, my colleagues and I observed the potential for modifiability within the child—whether minimal, moderate or considerable—we sought to create the psychological conditions for the parents to join us in an exciting and potentially exhilarating, challenging and, yes, at times disappointing process of moving into uncharted developmental waters for their child, beyond the presumed limitations of an autism diagnosis.

And so my ultimate goal in a first session was to bring the parents on board, to help them see the reasons why an ASD diagnosis, overgeneralized as it can be, should not be considered a definition of their child's being or a determinant of their child's future. There is room for action and for hope. I acknowledged openly that as a psychologist I could not promise results. Rather, I suggested that we embark together on a positive, optimistic dynamic way of working and allow the child's latent abilities—observed in tiny islets of normalcy which we would try to nurture—and not the diagnosis, lead the way.

By the end of several assessment sessions, my hope was that parents were beginning to understand that an autism diagnosis is not the sum total or the definition of who their child is. Evidence of symptoms serves us just as our operational baseline, so to speak, not in behavioral analysis terms but in dynamic terms: where did we start and what are we working *toward*? It is not simply the presence or absence of a symptom, I explained to parents, which is relevant, but a myriad of qualitative factors surrounding each symptom: its prevalence in the child's profile, its degree of intransigence, the possible precipitators, the level and kind of playful, creative energy needed to begin to transform it and, especially, its degree of modifiability when playfully or cognitively encountered. These considerations applied no matter how serious or pervasive the symptom constellation appeared at first.

It is important to point out that routinely I assured parents that, yes, I had noticed the symptomatic behavior that worried them and which had likely led to the purported diagnosis—such as poor eye contact, rigidity in or paucity of verbal communication, and/or stereotypical behaviors. Without this proviso, parents might have thought that I disagreed with the autism diagnosis, or the degree of its severity, simply because I had failed to see the child's problems. So the tone of a first session was often: "Yes, I see your child's difficulties. But I have also observed more than that."

Assuming that some parental discouragement had dissipated and that the parents had warmed to an alternative conceptualization of how their child's difficulties could be perceived and worked with—strength-focused and not diagnosis-focused—it was then important to introduce parents to the concept of islets of normalcy and their developmental significance. I wanted them to understand the necessity of identifying, expanding and strengthening these islets of normalcy and the positive role that they as parents could play in this process (as per Chapter 12). Because the identification and elicitation of islets of normalcy rests on a process of adult-child interaction and on the encounter with symptoms to tease out strengths, it was not enough to provide parents with theory. I wanted them to leave the office equipped with some practical tools.

And so the third element that helped to catalyze so many of the dramatic changes that we saw in children was parental consultation, that is, providing guidance, strategies and recommendations attuned to the profile of each child. Ideally, even by the end of a first session, I hoped that the parents would be open to receiving our recommendations regarding play and communication as well as many other strategies, "homework," some based on seeking islets of normalcy, others on creating circles of communication, and others based on developing early communication and learning skills. I sought to provide parents with developmentally sound and uncomplicated strategies that they could begin to apply with their child immediately. But suggesting to parents *what* to do, without first easing them from any resignation or discouragement, doubt or skepticism, all too often encountered, would have been futile. Parents have to see and feel that there are coherent reasons for letting their child's latent potential lead the way, rather than a diagnosis.

Usually the guidance I gave to parents focused on encouraging their alertness to islets of normalcy in their child, and on providing them with play strategies based on DIRFloortime to strengthen these islets. I also offered them ideas about how to encourage the development of imitation skills, mirror play for example, and guidelines related to communication, such as how to speak to their child and the importance of generous soliloquy.

Clearly, all three aspects—suspension of the overpowering influence of the diagnosis, shifting to a focus on islets of normalcy, and practical intervention strategies and recommendations—could not be addressed with parents in a single two-hour session. That is why several assessment sessions and subsequent follow-up sessions were so important, both to support the parents in the process of making a paradigm shift and to recalibrate recommendations and advice as the child improved. Not all parents remained with us longer term, as some of the stories in this book reflect. These stories were nevertheless featured because the impact of the three key elements of parental support catalyzed dramatic initial results, sometimes even within a short period.

Comprehensive Recommendations

The concept of practical, feasible homework for tired, busy and often over-whelmed parents included, on a per-case basis, a range of eclectic, far-reaching recommendations. There was significant overlap among the tips, pointers and strategies that were shared with nearly all parents of children thought to be autistic, particularly recommendations that pertained to communication strategies (especially the technique of soliloquy), play strategies, cognitive development strategies, the development of imitation skills and ideas for nurturing islets of normalcy. Other recommendations, given according to individual need, might include traditional therapies such as speech therapy, occupational therapy, physiotherapy, cranial-sacral physiotherapy, music therapy and referral to a DIR specialist for more intensive parent-child play work. (Practical pointers related to these recommendations can be found in Appendix III.)

Further individualized recommendations encompassed as many developmental areas and resources as appeared relevant and which could potentially advance each child's situation: teaching a child to read in order to build language through the visual channel; a neurological workup to rule out suspected neurological difficulties, particularly if any soft signs had been observed; a hearing test; referral to a doctor or to a licensed, reputable alternative medical specialist to dry up ear fluids; testing for casein, gluten or other food sensitivities; therapeutic gymnastics; play dates with typical peers; and many more. My underlying premise was that all channels of communication and functioning needed to be open, healthy and working well to achieve maximum progress, particularly with children whose symptoms presented as more stubborn or complex.

Relevant recommendations were prioritized and presented to parents selectively. There is a phenomenon known as "overtreatment" in which the young child is perpetually in a state of "being repaired." It was important to provide the parents with recommendations progressively, in response to the child's needs and rate of progress and the parents' own realities, in order not to overwhelm the child or the parents.

To summarize: helping parents see that a formal autism diagnosis does not need to spell developmental doom, enlightening them about the presence of islets of normalcy, offering them practical play and communication strategies which even a pressured parent could begin to do with the child, and providing them with essential and far-reaching recommendations in an attempt to approximate optimal conditions for developmental progress made a difference in hundreds of lives.

All of this transpired, it should be emphasized, with a very realistic eye to the fact that commonly in Israel both parents work long, hard hours, with the financial reality of the average family usually stressed. Time, energy and the financial resources to support the ideal greenhouse growth conditions were usually limited. Yet time and again, parents showed remarkable courage and determination in adopting our alternative, unconventional paradigm to help their child, with results so often encouraging and positive.

Educational Inclusion: A Key Recommendation

Although integrated, inclusive educational settings do exist in Israel, as discussed throughout this casebook, for the most part Israeli children who present with special needs are routinely placed in special education settings among similarly impaired children, in homogenous classes according to diagnosis. Therefore, as alluded to in other chapters, Israeli practitioners routinely recommend "communication kindergartens" for children thought to be autistic, "language kindergartens" for communication-impaired children with a non-autistic appearing profile, special schools for children with more challenging and complex autism-related problems, or special classrooms in regular schools for higher-functioning children with milder autistiform symptoms. While administratively this may have the advantage of centralizing therapeutic services for special needs children, developmentally and educationally there are serious weaknesses in such a system.

Children suspected of being autistic by definition suffer from some type of social communication problem. They are therefore in need of an educational environment which is rich in opportunities for typical peer modeling of language, play and learning skills. Placed in a special setting among communication- and socially-impaired peers, such children will find themselves in an environment where they receive several hours of speech and occupational therapy per week but lack typical peers with whom to interact. And so, attention to the type of educational setting was always a critical part of our recommendation process. I often recommended that younger children transfer as soon as possible from a special setting to an integrated educational setting, perhaps with the addition of speech or occupational therapies or Floortime to be provided by specialists privately. Older children, too, could benefit from inclusion but finding a setting where that was feasible was more challenging and entailed a lengthier search process.

If, as was often the case, integration through the system was not possible or the parents lacked the resources to create a tailor-made treatment program that included educational inclusion, then we lobbied for the child's placement in a special education setting among the highest functioning children that the educational system allowed. Often my colleagues and I sensed that the child's placement within an integrated setting, perhaps with an integration aide, would do wonders for the child's progress. However, the realities of the educational policies in Israel at the time often meant that children with more complex presentations would, nevertheless, be educated in special settings. We would then encourage the parents to seek opportunities to socially integrate their child with an aide in community center activity groups.

Swimming against the current of the commonly encountered policy of placement in special settings, and inspired by Feuerstein's conviction of the importance of a modifying environment to provide rich models for the child's imitation of fundamental developmental skills, my colleagues and I strongly advocated at municipal school placement meetings for the educational inclusion of children with suspected autism or other special needs. This was not a cookie-cutter, one-size-fits-all recommendation appropriate for every situation. However, having repeatedly witnessed the exciting benefits and the positive developmental impact of educational inclusion, we strongly favored this direction.

The long-term educational inclusion—which had been properly carried out—of Jack, Sasha, Annie, Davie, Josh and Ben, had helped propel these children over the developmental threshold into normative functioning.

A Potent Mix: Optimistic Attitude, Perceived Potential and Hard Work

My colleagues and I enjoyed remarkable and inspiring fruits of our labors as we witnessed gratifying progress among the children we assisted. For many of these children, their progress far exceeded what might have been expected given their presenting situation at the outset. It was not magic, but much hard work coupled with the vision of potential that brought about these changes. This hard work was inextricably bound to the optimistic Feuerstein theoretical outlook which assumed the intrinsic ability of the human being to change. It focused on the islets of normalcy which needed to be expanded and, as much as humanly possible, spared no effort to try to help each child, teen and adult achieve maximum potential.

Professor Feuerstein often liked to refer to himself as a "pathological optimist." This prompts a question: Doesn't an optimistic attitude toward autistiform behavior, which deemphasizes biological factors and emphasizes environmental variables, namely the human input, run the risk of causing parents to hope and then perhaps plummet into further disappointment? Parents yearn to believe in their child's potential. But many have endured so much distress in their child's early years that, understandably, they fear to adopt a more hopeful paradigm. Perhaps it is asking too much of a parent despondent about an autism diagnosis to embrace a little hope about the possibility of another outlook?

This is a question that I have discussed with many parents, in an effort to encourage them toward a paradigm shift—assuming, of course, that during dynamic assessment sessions I have first perceived the latent potential within their child. I give voice to their dilemma of feeling caught between a sense of resignation and their fear of being bitterly disappointed should they adopt a more flexible, optimistic way of working, with more positive expectations for their child. It can be frightening and potentially painful to hope for change and thus to risk disappointment.

There is a particular metaphor which often speaks to those parents caught between the hesitation to hope and the desire to hope: a sharp picket fence. Sitting on it hurts! The fence lies between two fields: on one side, a hopeful, more positive prognosis for their child, yet fraught with uncertainty. How do I know that my child will improve? Perhaps he or she is hopelessly unchangeable? On the other side, a less favorable prognosis, perhaps lower expectations, perhaps a sense of resignation, yet without the stress that the uncertainty of hope entails. It would be easier, in a sense, to slide off that painful fence of dilemma, and to drop down into the certainty of a deterministic diagnosis, even if it comes with a more negative prognosis.

I frankly admit to parents that by shifting their perspective and methods of working no one can promise that their child will progress normally or nearly so. *However*, if in the course of the initial assessment sessions my colleagues and I have been able to demonstrate to the parents that their child exhibits previously unseen or unappreciated islets of normalcy, and/or within the session there emerged subtle, often more than subtle, evidence of modifiability, we will then help the parents to internalize a more positive perspective, and support them by giving them tools for making certain changes in their approach to and interactions with their child.

Situations in which I was not able to bring my early glimpses of a child's latent potential to a satisfying level of realization left me feeling saddened and disappointed, in myself primarily, as to "what might have been." Perhaps I had failed in explaining to the parents the deep significance and wonderful promise that the tiniest islets of normalcy can portend? Perhaps I had not invested enough energy in helping the parents understand that their child's situation was not hopeless? Professor Feuerstein demanded maximum effort from his staff to help each child realize the potential he perceived. He often reminded us: "If you point to a child and find yourself thinking, 'the child can't do this, the child can't do that,' just look at your pointing hand! You will see that three of your fingers are pointing right back at yourself." The message to his staff was clear: to get better results, work harder!

Parent and Child Together

During dynamic assessment and follow-up sessions, it was not enough to discern the child's potential, to ascertain the intensity and complexity of symptoms, to elicit and encourage the child's latent strengths, and to demonstrate intervention strategies that worked, which the parents could then apply at home. It was also necessary to be sensitive to the energy, the time and the emotional and practical resources that were feasible for the parents to invest (alluded to above and in Chapter 12). As I played on the floor or worked at the table with a child, aside from the details of the child's difficulties and the child's strengths, I also wanted to supplement my overall impression of the general complexity of the child's problems with my impression of the emotional energy and practical resources of the parents.

In general, the children could be said to fall into three very loose, informal groupings. In the first grouping were children with suspected autism whose presentations were normal or nearly normal. They displayed many islets of normalcy, they engaged with their parents or with me relatively readily, and I felt confident that, despite any developmental idiosyncrasies, they would thrive in educationally inclusive settings, with the possible addition of some individual therapies.

In the second grouping were children whose profiles were more challenging, yet nevertheless promising. Their islets of normalcy were less prevalent, and these sparser islets might require greater effort and creativity to elicit. But the dynamic, interactive assessment sessions nevertheless had shown that, with an investment of focused energy and an application of our recommendations, substantive change was possible. The child would require more intensive intervention and more follow-up sessions than children in the first grouping, and parents would require more guidance in order to attain the positive prognosis perceived. If parents had the financial means, I usually referred such children for additional private therapies, which varied widely on a per-case basis, for more intensive developmental treatment. The child's acceptance into an inclusive educational setting, usually with an aide in order to pull the child's functioning toward the norm, was usually critical for this middle group of moderately challenged children. The developmental prognosis appeared positive.

In the third loose grouping, the child's islets of normalcy were few and required more intense effort to reveal them. These more seriously challenged children often, but not always, presented with entrenched symptoms, usually compounded by verified genetic, neurological and/or physiological problems, giving them additional degrees of challenge and complexity. Challenge and complexity, yes. Hopelessness, no.

There was not a single person whom Reuven Feuerstein considered hopeless or impervious to change. The notion of "hopeless" was not part of his lexicon or that of his staff. The children who presented with a high degree of complexity would likely require more frequent follow-ups at the Institute, a more intensive program of private therapies, recommendations for medical clarifications and more intensive parental guidance.

In situations where autistiform symptoms occurred concurrently with physiological challenges, such as a genetic syndrome or neurological problems, the level of parental discouragement was usually deep and intense. Often other practitioners had communicated to these parents a sense of hopelessness regarding the prognosis of their child. Inspired by Feuerstein's clinical wisdom and experience across several generations, my colleagues and I endeavored to help parents understand that while normative performance might not prove to be feasible—although we would aim for it!—meaningful change and improvement were still options even with complex and challenging developmental problems.

These three loose groupings were not part of any scoring or diagnostic system, nor were they discussed with parents. These groupings served me as a mental guide and a reminder of the intensity and scope of input, energy, information, emotional support, guidance and recommendations that the parents would need to receive at the Institute in order to help actualize their child's potential maximally.

So in those early appointments when working with the child, I also attempted to ascertain the degree of parental openness to our perspective, willingness to apply our recommendations, energy and resources that were needed and/or available to embark on a paradigm shift for their child. Usually not expressed aloud, the following questions were held in mind: How discouraged did the parents appear? What information did they require to help soothe their discouragement and help them galvanize their energy toward a different way of perceiving and helping their child? Were both parents working? Would either parent be able to find or make the time to play with the child and/or take the child to additional therapies? Were the parents open to follow-up appointments at the Institute? Were they open to parent consults? Were the parents prepared and able to apply practical tools for enhancing their child's developmental strengths that were based on a mixture of Feuerstein's methods intertwined with Floortime play strategies for enhancing communication and relationship? Did the parents have the financial means to provide any therapies privately? Was the child placed in a setting that could stimulate progress? Was the child in an educational setting where the staff was open to our ideas and recommendations?

I wish that I could say that I had developed an algorithm that produced correlation coefficients to answer a question like: Would a child with mild autistiform symptoms but whose parents were deeply discouraged progress better than a child with more serious symptoms but whose parents were energetic and eager to try our suggestions? But an algorithm was not the purpose of the exercise. My aim was always to simultaneously weigh the child's strengths and weaknesses while remaining sensitive to the level of parents' emotional resilience versus discouragement, openness versus resistance to our way of working and the availability of time and other resources their child might require. A parent's degree of discouragement or level of resistance to a new way of thinking did not necessarily prevent the work from continuing. The genuine answers to these questions helped me remain sensitive to the complex dynamic before me and to attune many aspects of my work to the needs and the strengths of the parents and child as a unit.

Reports as Educational Tools

At the end of each assessment session, I shared with the parents a verbal description of my initial observations of their child, pointing out the child's islets of normalcy and their significance, and providing them with recommendations for enhancing the child's progress. There were no scores, only qualitative descriptions, unique for each child.

Our written reports did not aim to deliver a diagnosis, as in conventional assessment, but rather an insightful blueprint for change. Beyond detailing our observations and impressions of a child's functioning, we wanted our reports to serve as educational tools, for parents and for other practitioners, in explaining how the dynamic paradigm affords not only an alternative vision of the child's capacities but also stimulates the production of practical ideas and strategies for realizing that vision.

In situations where we concurred with previous reports that the child was genuinely autistic, our written dynamic report related first of all to the perceived accuracy of the diagnosis, *but* then fully elaborated our efforts to change the child's presentation, with special attention to what worked. In artificially brief form for purposes of example, such a report might sound something like: "Harry initially presented with an intense degree of emotional cutoffness, rocking silently in the corner with his back to me, as he waved a marker in front of his eyes. While his presentation appeared to fit classic autism diagnostic criteria, after roughly an hour of his silent, aloof rocking, a number of play strategies, some derived from Floortime, helped to penetrate his isolation ... These strategies included placing a mirror in front of him so that his occasional glancing up guaranteed a flash of eye contact, gently holding him and rocking with him as I attempted to pat his feet .... In this initial two-hour session, with several other assessment sessions to follow, I noticed that Harry responds to soft music. He stopped rocking when I hummed to him .... Although his initial presentation appeared worrisome, initial play-based forays into contact and communication with Harry yielded glimmers of eye contact and eventually a little smile of pleasure when he leaned back into my arms and stopped rocking. Interim recommendations for enhancing contact with Harry include ..."

In our reports for children whose formal diagnoses of presumed autism, PDD-NOS or "spectrum" were found to be inaccurate or misleading, we took a stand. We first acknowledged the diagnosis that the child had received elsewhere, and then we discussed how we had reached the conclusion that the original autism diagnosis was inaccurate. This was done by highlighting the child's observed functional strengths and by explaining why, in our estimation, the autism diagnosis did not apply. A report for such a child might sound something like: "Jesse was diagnosed with Autistic Spectrum Disorder two months ago at the Child Developmental Clinic of a Major Hospital .... However, in our interactive, dynamic assessment of Jesse, using the following play-based learning materials ... Jesse displayed an excellent sense of humor, readily engaged with the assessor and participated with sincere interest in age-appropriate cognitive activities which required dialogue with the assessor. Jesse's mother revealed the traumatic loss of his paternal grandfather three months ago, leading to his disturbed sleep problems and bedwetting. It would appear that Jesse's more withdrawn presentation several months ago reflected his traumatic loss. We have concluded that the autism diagnosis does not apply in his situation and recommend that ..."

What of the Many Other Children?

My general records showed that over the years the Institute received on average between fifty to one hundred *new* referrals of children annually who had been diagnosed elsewhere as autistic, in addition to those whose progress was already being followed by us. If I do the math for a career of twenty-five years, then we are talking about several thousand children with autistiform symptoms who passed through our offices, in addition to many hundreds, likely thousands, of other children who presented with an enormous array of other diagnoses and conditions. This book tells largely of significant, pivotal assessment and early treatment experiences which led to rewarding fuller stories for most, though not all, of these fourteen children. What of the many hundreds more children with suspected autism whom my colleagues and I saw? What are the outlines of their stories, too many to be told, with their details now archived in dusty boxes? Were these fourteen children the only ones to enjoy a dramatic jumpstart to their development? Hardly.

Deep in the trenches, assiduously focusing on the task of detecting potential within complex presentations, identifying strengths within even the most challenged child, and then emotionally and practically supporting the parents to work toward those strengths within a broader educational system that, to our dismay, relied on diagnoses and often highlighted deficiencies, I did not have the luxury of time to create a statistical base to corroborate memory. I can only share with readers my recollection of the overall impact of our working positively and dynamically for many years with children thought to be autistic, but whose stories could not be told in this book. It can be safely said that my colleagues and I almost always made a positive difference. But what does this mean in a practical sense?

Very few children failed to change in some degree or to improve at all. In such cases, like Amy (Chapter 12), the child's presentation was so complex and challenging that the process of identifying and eliciting islets of normalcy, confirming the child's latent abilities, and working toward change required more time to allow fragile, early changes to take root, more follow-up visits to the Institute, more parental support to enable the fragile islets of normalcy to take hold in her profile, and more time, energy and financial resources to provide supplemental therapies than were realistically possible for the parents.

In a relative minority of situations, improvements were token or short-lived, especially if the child's development was left unsupported by follow-up appointments with us, additional therapies were not feasible and/or the child's educational setting was not adequate. In a slightly larger minority, the developmental improvements we facilitated were modest, minimal, and hard-won over time, particularly when the symptom presentations were complex, or were complicated by other developmental conditions, such as genetic syndromes or physiological impairments. Yet even with these children, we worked full out to find and elicit those precious islets of normalcy and to encourage deeply discouraged parents to dare to raise the bar of expectations regarding their child's abilities and prognosis.

More frequently, improvements were moderate and fairly stable, and strengths began to predominate in the child's profile. Very often, progress was dramatic and significant, with changes that were long-lasting and well-stabilized in the child's profile. There were also some children whose significant progress in early childhood later weakened in the face of developmental crises, such as puberty, family tensions or, as in the case of Ernie (Chapter 10), when the system suddenly curtailed the child's educational inclusion.

Limited progress in a child might be traced to myriad reasons that were rooted in the complex interplay among the intensity and complexity of a child's presenting problems, the child's latent strengths, and the combined practical resources of the educational system and the family. Sometimes I considered the reason to lie in a self-perceived failure on my part to reach and engage the parents, especially if they held tight to a model of working with their child which doubted that fundamental change was possible with autism. In some cases, the parents had found a sense of certainty in an autism diagnosis, which gave them a term which appeared to offer clarity, thus ending for them a stressful period of uncertainty as to "what's wrong with my child?" I never judged these parents, as the stress on parents is always great. To embrace another way of looking at their child might mean reopening a painful wound. But my colleagues and I always felt saddened when we saw the potential of the child behind the autistiform symptoms yet we were not able to persuade the parents that there is another way of perceiving their child and advancing his or her potential progress.

Fortunately, overall my colleagues and I can look back on a rewarding period of significant help to many children and their parents, inspired by the clinical insights and the courage of the late Professor. We can recall assessment sessions in which parents broke down in tears of joy when they understood that there was genuine hope for their child. We can recall many intense meetings guiding and counseling parents, and then the encouraging follow-up sessions when these parents told us that they had attempted, despite their doubts, to adopt our recommendations, with positive results. We can recall many parents who phoned years later to share with us wonderful news of their child's progress since they had last visited the Institute. Many, even most, but—we must be candid—not all. That is the reality of this demanding yet satisfying work.

Practitioners as Positive Partners

When parents or practitioners working with children presenting with autistiform symptoms adopt and internalize the attitude that significant modifiability is possible, they will not approach autism as a terminal condition from which meaningful change could never evolve but rather will view the autistiform symptoms as a starting point from which meaningful developmental change can ensue. Sometimes, the child before us presents with an overwhelming sense of impairment and *apparently* intransigent symptoms. The fact that genuinely autistic children can present difficult challenges does not mean that they lack the capacity for modifiability. When we conclude so, we may only be acknowledging our own sense of frustration or of failure with them, which I have naturally experienced as well.

There is no need, however, to project our frustration and discouragement onto a child who appears to be autistic. If we do so, we run the risk of prematurely foreclosing our therapeutic efforts, limiting these efforts to the confines of our discouraged vision. When we internalize the notion that the human being is inherently modifiable, we are inspired to persevere in our efforts to bring about changes, which at first may be so subtle as to be practically microscopic. With modifiability as a watchword, the practitioner will not conclude, as is all too common in the field today, that the child with autistiform symptoms is necessarily destined to a life of restricted functioning.

My colleagues and I never falsely promised change or assured parents that every child thought to be autistic would achieve normative functioning. Rather, we worked with the expectation that the propensity for modifiability is part of the human condition, that these children can positively benefit from this worldview, and that we must spare no effort in trying to help the child reach his or her maximum potential, whether that maximum ultimately extends into a normative range or not.

Revisiting Kanner

While writing the conclusion for this casebook, I decided to revisit Leo Kanner's summaries of the eleven case studies with which he first introduced his concept of early infantile autism.[3] Later, over the course of a generation or so, he compiled at least one hundred representative cases. But I was intrigued by the descriptions of these first eleven children. Each child was unique in his or her presentation. At the same time, there were commonalities, to a degree, among their various symptoms: idiosyncratic, mechanical language; mutism; lack of use of the first-person pronoun; incoherent speech; seeing people as unwelcome intruders; social isolation; a sense of being emotionally unreachable; limited affective contact; resistance to interpersonal contact; obsessive repetitive behaviors; distress at disruptions of routines or changes in objects and so on. Kanner described a range of presentations, perhaps what could even be considered a spectrum—the very term I have found to be so problematic for so many children!

However, looking closely at the way in which Kanner gradually honed in on the criteria he considered primary for identifying an autistic condition, I noticed that his diagnostic criteria were anything but general, elastic or spectrum inducing. He spoke of "extreme autistic aloneness," "profound aloneness," "extreme autism, obsessiveness, stereotypy and echolalia," "impenetrable aloneness, "an anxiously obsessive desire for the maintenance of sameness," "a peculiar type of obsessiveness." Ultimately, Kanner focused on two primary symptoms: "extreme isolation and obsessive insistence on sameness."[4] He also cited secondary symptoms, such as fascination with objects, and impaired or idiosyncratic verbal communication. But pointedly, it appears that Kanner considered that any manifestations in his two core symptom areas had to be extreme, profound and/or obsessive.

This emphasis on *extreme* symptomatology is a far cry from where we are today in the consideration and diagnosis of autism. Currently, for example, children who have difficulty initiating a conversation, who are reluctant to engage in reciprocal play activities or who insist on the same morning routine, risk being quickly pegged as autistic. The net of the autism diagnosis has been stretched so widely that, as the stories in this casebook reflect, it appears to have lost its clinical essence and diagnostic power.

Using the term "autistiform" to describe behaviors that remind us of autism could go a long way toward helping to prevent the misdiagnosis and/or misinterpretation of mild to moderate developmental challenges in many children. I also believe that it would be preferable to return to Kanner's more restricted primary criteria—and even to go beyond that, to use a stringent interpretation of Kanner's two primary criteria. The stories of the children in this casebook hopefully persuade us to save the term "autism" for the most extreme presentations that suit Kanner's two criteria and to apply the term "autistic" most cautiously.

And what shall we call the other children, those who present with milder manifestations of social communication challenges and idiosyncratic behaviors? Above all, we will call them children, some perhaps with mild and reversible developmental difficulties, others for whom a functional description will suffice, others with conditions for which an alternative understanding and/or diagnosis may more accurately shed light on their difficulties, and yet others who need just a little more time and perhaps some skilled support to attain normative or near normative functioning. And if we cannot fit a child's condition into the confines of a diagnostic category then, certainly, concentrating on understanding a child's developmental predicament and focusing our energies on helping the child find a way out of that predicament is a satisfying way of working with the challenge of suspected autism.

Kanner's cases from over seventy years ago intrigued me. As I reread his case vignettes, I could not help wondering how the parents of those eleven children might have responded to Feuerstein's belief in the capacity for modifiability, how each child might have changed in response to the warm, developmentally-attuned play strategies of DIRFloortime, what islets of normalcy might have been created and, simply, what might have been.

The Children Speak

And the children who featured in this casebook, what might they say about the changes they underwent? Perhaps ...

Jack: "I never was autistic. I'm a bit shy socially, and not at the top of my class. But inside, I'm a warm, lively kid and fun to play with. Please keep believing in me."

Sasha: "I was stuck and not at all with it when I was baby. Luckily my parents found a speech therapist who knew wonderful play activities that helped me connect with myself and with others. I love school and my friends."

Annie: "I was so anxious when I was two years old. And I didn't like it when my little brother was born either. It was a tough journey, but being with kids who talked and played normally helped a lot. My parents used to worry that I was autistic. I'm so glad that they started to feel happier and believe in my potential when they saw all the progress I began to make. They relaxed a lot. School is fun. I love having friends."

Davie: "It's true I still toe-walk a bit when I feel tense. But I've got lots of friends at school. They like me, and I like them. Pokémon and his buddies are really cool."

Joe: "I'm doing a lot better now than I was a few years ago. I guess some people would see me as a little different because my communication skills are not on par with my age. I'm really enjoying my program for youth with special needs. I understand more than people think I do!"

Mikey: "I'm glad my mom started to talk to me. I didn't even care about what. Just the fact that she talked to me helped me a lot. I wish we could have kept going to the Institute. It was different there."

Max: "I was so frustrated because I understood so much but I couldn't get my mouth, lips and tongue to make the sounds I needed. Life got better when I got special help on how to use my mouth muscles so I could talk. I'm pretty smart."

Josh: "Was I ever a scared little kid! I was so overwhelmed that I could hardly talk. Some people even thought I was autistic. I remember that some lady played with me and we made a wonderful mess throwing toys around. Slowly things got a lot better. Too busy to add more. I'm getting ready for a date."

Working dynamically—putting the diagnosis aside, eschewing the tallying of symptoms and the reliance on official generalized criteria in favor of personalized descriptions, seeking and emphasizing the child's latent strengths, nurturing those strengths so that they gradually overcome the impact of initial difficulties—is a truly wonderful, satisfying and effective way of working with children with autistiform symptoms. For many practitioners, working with these children qualitatively, descriptively and playfully, rather than quantitatively with normed instruments in search of a formal diagnosis, takes them beyond their comfort zone. I hope that in some small but meaningful way this book will strengthen practitioners to edge toward the kind of paradigm shift this book embraces and that it will encourage parents to believe more in the potential than the presumed pathology of their child. There are many wonderful children behind autistiform symptoms just waiting.

Notes

1 Serena Wieder, personal communication to author (January 10, 2020). The observation was made by Dr. Wieder at a small training seminar, whose precise date proved untraceable; point clarified in personal communication.

2 Louis H. Falik, *Changing Destinies: The Life and Times of Prof. Reuven Feuerstein* (Bloomington, IN: Xlibris, 2019), 275.

3 Leo Kanner, "Autistic Disturbances of Affective Contact," *Nervous Child* 2 (1943): 217–50.

4 Leo Kanner, *Childhood Psychosis: Initial Studies and New Insights* (Washington, DC: Winston, 1973).

References

Falik, Louis H. *Changing Destinies: The Life and Times of Prof. Reuven Feuerstein.* Bloomington, IN: Xlibris, 2019.

Kanner, Leo. "Autistic Disturbances of Affective Contact." *Nervous Child* 2 (1943): 217–50.

Kanner, Leo. *Childhood Psychosis: Initial Studies and New Insights.* Washington, DC: Winston, 1973.

Appendix I

DSM-IV-TR **Diagnostic Criteria for Autistic Disorder
299.00**

A. A total of six (or more) items from (1), (2), and (3), with at least two from
    (1), and one each from (2) and (3):

    (1) Qualitative impairment in social interaction, as manifested by at least
        two of the following:

        (a) marked impairment in the use of multiple nonverbal behaviors
            such as eye-to-eye gaze, facial expression, body postures, and
            gestures to regulate social interaction
        (b) failure to develop peer relationships appropriate to developmental
            level
        (c) a lack of spontaneous seeking to share enjoyment, interests or
            achievements with other people (e.g., by a lack of showing,
            bringing or pointing out objects of interest)
        (d) lack of social or emotional reciprocity

    (2) Qualitative impairments in communication as manifested by at least
        one of the following:

        (a) delay in, or total lack of, the development of spoken language
            (not accompanied by an attempt to compensate through
            alternative modes of communication such as gesture or mime)
        (b) in individuals with adequate speech, marked impairment in the
            ability to initiate or sustain a conversation with others
        (c) stereotyped and repetitive use of language or idiosyncratic
            language
        (d) lack of varied, spontaneous, make-believe play or social imitative
            play appropriate to developmental level

    (3) Restricted, repetitive and stereotyped patterns of behavior, interests
        and activities, as manifested by at least one of the following:

(a) encompassing preoccupation with one or more stereotyped and restricted patterns of interest that is abnormal either in intensity or focus

(b) apparently inflexible adherence to specific nonfunctional routines or rituals

(c) stereotyped and repetitive motor mannerisms (e.g., hand or finger flapping or twisting, or complex whole-body movements)

(d) persistent preoccupation with parts of objects

B. Delays or abnormal functioning in at least one of the following areas, with onset prior to age three years: (1) social interaction, (2) language as used in social communication, or (3) symbolic or imaginative play.

C. The disturbance is not better accounted for by Rett's Disorder or Childhood Disintegrative Disorder.

Reprinted with permission from the Diagnostic and Statistical Manual of Mental Disorders, Fourth Edition Text Revision (Copyright ©2000). American Psychiatric Association. All Rights Reserved.

Appendix II

DSM-5 Criteria for Autistic Spectrum Disorder 299.00 (F84.0)

A. Persistent deficits in social communication and social interaction across multiple contexts, as manifested by the following, currently or by history (examples are illustrative, not exhaustive, see text):

1. Deficits in social-emotional reciprocity, ranging, for example, from abnormal social approach and failure of normal back-and-forth conversation; to reduced sharing of interests, emotions, or affect; to failure to initiate or respond to social interactions.
2. Deficits in nonverbal communicative behaviors used for social interaction, ranging, for example, from poorly integrated verbal and nonverbal communication; to abnormalities in eye contact and body language or deficits in understanding and use of gestures; to a total lack of facial expressions and nonverbal communication.
3. Deficits in developing, maintaining, and understanding relationships, ranging, for example, from difficulties adjusting behavior to suit various social contexts; to difficulties in sharing imaginative play or in making friends; to absence of interest in peers.

Specify current severity: **Severity is based on social communication impairments and restricted repetitive patterns of behavior**. (See Table 1.)

B. Restricted, repetitive patterns of behavior, interests, or activities, as manifested by at least two of the following, currently or by history (examples are illustrative, not exhaustive; see text):

1. Stereotyped or repetitive motor movements, use of objects, or speech (e.g., simple motor stereotypies, lining up toys or flipping objects, echolalia, idiosyncratic phrases).
2. Insistence on sameness, inflexible adherence to routines, or ritualized patterns of verbal or nonverbal behavior (e.g., extreme distress at

small changes, difficulties with transitions, rigid thinking patterns, greeting rituals, need to take same route or eat same food every day).

3. Highly restricted, fixated interests that are abnormal in intensity or focus (e.g., strong attachment to or preoccupation with unusual objects, excessively circumscribed or perseverative interest).

4. Hyper- or hyporeactivity to sensory input or unusual interests in sensory aspects of the environment (e.g., apparent indifference to pain/temperature, adverse response to specific sounds or textures, excessive smelling or touching of objects, visual fascination with lights or movement).

Specify current severity: **Severity is based on social communication impairments and restricted, repetitive patterns of behavior.** (See Table 1.)

C. Symptoms must be present in the early developmental period (but may not become fully manifest until social demands exceed limited capacities or may be masked by learned strategies in later life).

D. Symptoms cause clinically significant impairment in social, occupational, or other important areas of current functioning.

E. These disturbances are not better explained by intellectual disability (intellectual developmental disorder) or global developmental delay. Intellectual disability and autism spectrum disorder frequently co-occur; to make comorbid diagnoses of autism spectrum disorder and intellectual disability, social communication should be below that expected for general developmental level.

Note: Individuals with a well-established DSM-IV diagnosis of autistic disorder, Asperger's disorder, or pervasive developmental disorder not otherwise specified should be given the diagnosis of autism spectrum disorder. Individuals who have marked deficits in social communication, but whose symptoms do not otherwise meet criteria for autism spectrum disorder, should be evaluated for social (pragmatic) communication disorder.

Specify if:

With or without accompanying intellectual impairment
With or without accompanying language impairment
Associated with a known medical or genetic condition or environmental factor (Coding note: Use additional code to identify the associated medical or genetic condition.)
Associated with another neurodevelopmental, mental, or behavioral disorder (Coding note: Use additional code[s] to identify the associated neurodevelopmental, mental, or behavioral disorder[s].)

With catatonia (refer to the criteria for catatonia association with another mental disorder, pp. 119-120, for definition). (**Coding note:** Use additional code 293.89 [F06.1] catatonia associated with autism spectrum disorder to indicate the presence of the comorbid catatonia.)

[Table 1 is not reproduced here.]

Reprinted with permission from the Diagnostic and Statistical Manual of Mental Disorders, Fifth Edition (Copyright © 2013). American Psychiatric Association. All Rights Reserved.

Appendix III

Practical Points for Parents

Where do you go from here if you are a parent of a child thought to be autistic, or if you are a practitioner seeking to work in a paradigm outside the conventional box? Here are some suggestions that I have found to be most practical and helpful in jumpstarting the process of modifiability in children thought to be autistic. Obviously, these ideas do not offer instant solutions to developmental challenges. But over the years, they have helped many parents.

Each child is different and unique, so these ideas can't be applied to every child in cookie-cutter fashion. Many have been derived either from Feuerstein methodology or from DIRFloortime practice. These frequently recommended ideas proved to be doable for most parents. Often they yielded the first glimmers of promising change. Attunement is a key word—to the needs, abilities and sensitivities of each child. The following practical points have helped many parents.

Seek practitioners who see the potential in your child and who are committed to working to help your child realize his or her potential. There are many psychologists, psychiatrists, occupational and speech therapists, physiotherapists and teachers who intuitively or through training see the child behind the symptoms. Seek out therapists, educators and other practitioners who see your child and who believe in your child's strengths. An initially discouraging or pessimistic report of your child's abilities and prognosis may or may not be correct, or it may not reflect the whole picture. Or, a clinician's reading of your child's difficulties might be accurate, but that person might have overlooked your child's strengths, islets of normalcy, the evidence of your child's ability to change. It is important to see a child's problems or symptoms, but it is even more important to see a child's potential and to offer recommendations to realize that potential. The diagnosis itself should not be given the power to determine your child's future. Seek out professionals who see your child behind the symptoms.

Become a super-sleuth in identifying your child's islets of normalcy. You will be looking for increasingly warmer and more sustained eye contact, evidence that your child is showing signs of nonverbal connection, gestures, babbling and then syllables and words, a sense of humor, growing pleasure and delight in physical and emotional contact, evidence of anticipation, enthusiasm for activities, turn-taking interest and abilities, growing interest in symbolic and pretend play, and any other behaviors that typify normative functioning.

Delight in these islets when you see them and treasure their developmental importance. Use playfully interactive strategies to help these islets grow and consolidate. Qualified DIR professionals can assist you in this process.

Talk to your child. Despite your child's lack of language or difficulties with verbal communication, don't assume that he or she does not understand. Most children understand more than they are able to express. I have found that it is preferable not to pressure the child or try to squeeze language from the child but to create an environment that warmly encourages the desire for the child to speak.

About what should you speak? Talk to, or even at, your child or simply aloud to yourself in the presence of your child, about what is happening, what happened, and/or what is going to happen. Talk about things outside the child (surroundings, events) or inside the child (feelings). While the exercises that your child's speech therapist recommends require your child's attention, soliloquies are meant to be relaxed, without demanding the child's attention. Just let your language flow.

A typical soliloquy might sound like: "Now where did I put my keys? I need to go to the store to get some milk for breakfast tomorrow. Daddy is home, and he'll watch you while I'm gone. Bye for now."

Or: "Time to get dressed. This light blue shirt looks just right with your corduroy pants. I'm helping you with your right arm first, now your left. Only four buttons, one, two, three, and four. You look so handsome."

Or as father lifts the child who may not even be looking at daddy: "Up you come. I'm going to lift you way up high and oops! One, two, three—up! I caught you. Now it's tickle time. Don't worry, I'll be gentle."

Or: "You're so sad. You were running fast and fell down. It's not fair, is it? It's not fun to get hurt." Even in the car, you can talk about the traffic or what you notice along the way.

At first, you may literally feel as if you are talking to the wall, especially if your child is not responding or showing signs of attending. Try not to get discouraged, and keep going. The purpose of soliloquy is to immerse your child in an ocean of spoken language. Continue to talk plentifully to your child about what is going on, without exhausting yourself. It can make a difference over time.

Consider the following. If parents assume, or have been told, that their child isn't interested in verbal communication or is incapable of understanding speech, and the parents have stopped talking to the child, the child might feel left in his or her own world with the feeling that there is no one out there. By speaking a lot to, at or simply in the presence of your child—without demanding a response or even attention—you communicate your presence and send out a message of connection to your child. This surround sound gradually warms up the receptive language channel. It creates an awareness of sounds and a sense of connection with others, later an interest in listening—all preparing the groundwork toward speech. This "at-home" surround sound can be a wonderful complement to the efforts of your child's speech therapist.

You might feel skeptical at first of the value of talking "at," to or nearby your child. But many parents have given us encouraging feedback, such as the child's improved eye contact, more babbling, more words, or the child's stronger emotional presence.

Don't force your child to look at you as you speak in soliloquy fashion. When you want your child's eye contact, seek out his or her gaze yourself. Bend down or move around to your child's line of vision. Make it playful. There are wonderful play-based strategies in DIR for warmly eliciting eye contact.

Speak slowly and clearly when you talk to your child. This makes it easier for your child to process what he or she hears. The clearer the messages going in to a child's brain, the less energy is wasted by the child in the frustrating task of deciphering/processing what has been said. That leaves more developmental energy for the child to attend, to take an interest in the world, or even to make those precious first babbling sounds or words—which you can then imitate or respond to.

If you have ever learned a foreign or a second language, you know how much more of that language you understand when someone takes the time to speak to you slowly and clearly. Write "speak slowly and clearly" and tape the note to your fridge as a reminder to slow down your speech. You should see an impact on your child over time.

Climb the DIR developmental ladder with your child. There are many trained, qualified professionals proficient in DIRFloortime. They can be of great assistance in guiding you to connect, communicate and play with your child.

Climb the related communication pyramid. At the base of the communication pyramid is the ability to receive and enjoy touch. Baby playtime, gentle tickling, rocking, holding your child in your lap facing you on the swing, and so on, can be helpful to lay the groundwork for communication. Communication starts with touch that is accepted and enjoyed by the child. The climb toward speech continues as you use playful strategies to build warmer, more consistent eye contact. DIR strategies will help you here too.

Warm accepted touch, along with eye contact, is what inspires infants to begin babbling, and these same ingredients are useful with the young child with autistic symptoms. With you talking more to your child and gently seeking out his or her eye contact, your child might just begin to vocalize or babble a little. That is good news because babbling is the raw material of speech. Children don't begin speaking in sentences. Start at the base of the communication pyramid with touch, build eye contact, and then enjoy imitating and responding verbally to your child's babbling or words.

Speak your child's language—babble back in response! Try not to let any sound, syllable, tune or word of a largely nonspeaking child go unanswered.

Always respond to your child's simple babbling or attempts at words. Imitate or just comment. Maintain the DIR circles of communication and the sense of reciprocity that Feuerstein speaks about.

As your child begins to show early communication abilities, gradually use an increasingly richer vocabulary with your child, and emphasize your spoken key words in context. Your verbal response strategies will change as your child moves from silence to babbling and, hopefully, beyond. Continue to speak slowly and clearly to help your child process. Over time, you will use increasingly longer sentences, a more developed vocabulary, and even concepts.

I often coached parents to keep their level of expressive language just above the level of the child's apparent comprehension and expressive language. The degree of "above" differs for each child. Your verbal feedback to your child might sound like, "Yes! Blue!" Or, "*First* we're going to the store, and *then* we're visiting *Gramma.*" Note that at this stage you are using language in context, while still speaking slowly and clearly; but now you are emphasizing key words within the sentence to aid your child in understanding.

Expand! This is a key DIR recommendation which means keep elaborating, and keep that sense of connection and communication going, whether during play, speech or activities of daily life. I sometimes added what I called the "One Two Three" rule. If your child is generally uttering one word at a time, then respond with two. Child: "Juice!" Mother: "Yummy juice." Similarly, if your child speaks in two-word utterances, then respond in three-word utterances until linguistic momentum improves. Child: "Big dog." Father: "Big furry dog!"

There is no hard and fast mathematical principle at work. The general idea is not to simply repeat the words your child said but to build on the child's every tiny step of progress and to increase the length and complexity of your responses accordingly.

Imitation! Enjoy frequent mirror play. Mirror play is a wonderful way to work on eye contact, sound, syllable and word production, and the key underlying developmental skill of imitation with young children.

With your young child seated on your lap as you both face a mirror which reflects your face and upper body, let your sensitivity and imagination run free as you engage in play that encourages any of the above developmental skills (eye contact, sound production etc.). You might gently tickle your child to encourage the child's gaze into the mirror. You want your eyes and your facial expression to communicate warmth and pleasure in contact.

If your child emits any sounds, syllables or words, speak your child's language and imitate them right back! If your child makes unintentional or purposeful head or hand movements, imitate these to create a conversation of imitated movement.

Perhaps gently cover the child's eyes with your hands to start a game of peek-a-boo, or throw a blanket over your head or the child's head to create mirrored drama and interaction. Wave your child's arms or rock gently as you sing a lovely rhythmic song that just might open some circles of communication and yield islets of normalcy.

You can draw from the playful, communication-enhancing ideas of DIRFloortime. That literature is full of playful ideas for creating circles of communication. Even ten minutes of mirror time once or twice a day can make a difference.

There are benefits to educational inclusion. Consult with professionals who believe in the developmental benefits and the positive impact of educational integration (inclusion), and who are able to create opportunities for inclusion best suited to your child. The readiness of the educational setting, the openness and confidence of the teacher, the existence of a support system for inclusion within the school, the possibility of an integration aide, the child's individual readiness for inclusion—all of these factors need to be weighed to ensure a promising inclusion experience. When "best practice" circumstances are not available for inclusion within the school system, often opportunities for social inclusion can be created in community center activity groups, youth groups, scout groups, day camps and so on. Proper inclusion requires supervision and consultation for the integration aide, when necessary, as well as professional guidance and support for the staff involved.

Be courageous in your struggle to trust your instincts and your understanding of your child's strengths. With time and practice, you will become more skilled in observing, eliciting and strengthening your child's islets of normalcy. These are windows into your child's capacities. Enjoy these moments, which hopefully will continue to accumulate and grow in your child's profile.

Dads, you are important and have lots to give to your child! Mothers often wept in my office, sometimes in distress over an autism diagnosis that other professionals had applied to their child, sometimes when they saw the first glimmers of hope, and sometimes when they began to see meaningful changes in their child. Fathers were usually less inclined to show their feelings. They often appeared stoic, but likely suffering within, not certain what they could do to help improve their child's situation. Fathers, the little things you do to play with, talk to or interact with your child can make a big difference over time. Some fathers are wonderful down on the floor, gently tickling the child or pushing tiny cars back and forth with the child. Others excel at rough-housing. Those strong movements of gently tossing, rocking or swinging the child can be so helpful in unlocking your child's pent-up tension, withheld vocalization (sounds) or even speech.

Sometimes I found that fathers' "extra demands at the office" were a reflection of their own sadness or feelings of discouragement in the face of their child's difficulties. I encourage dads to get playfully involved in spite of any lurking sadness or frustration related to the home situation. Your relationship with your child may be different from your spouse's, but your role is no less important. It takes a bit of practice to play with a child experiencing developmental challenges, but the rewards are great. I usually suggested that mothers not nag fathers to get involved with the child. Instead, *encourage* them, and give dad some good ideas of what to do and how to play. Try building into your talking time with your spouse the emotional safety, patience and noncritical attitude that makes it safe for each of you to talk about any feelings of frustration, discouragement, sadness that you might be feeling as you climb that developmental ladder with your child. Sometimes it's a challenging climb, but it's a worthwhile one.

Index